Clinical Hypnosis and Therapeutic Suggestion in Patient Care

Edited by

Rothlyn P. Zahourek
M.S., R.N., C.S.

BRUNNER / MAZEL, *Publishers* • New York

Library of Congress Cataloging-in-Publication Data
Clinical hypnosis and therapeutic suggestion in patient care / edited
by Rothlyn P. Zahourek.
    p.   cm.
  Reprint. Originally published: Orlando : Grune & Stratton, c1985.
  Includes bibliographical references.
  Includes index.
  1. Hypnotism—Therapeutic use. 2. Nursing. I. Zahourek, Rothlyn
P., 1943.
  [DNLM: 1. Hypnosis—patient care.   WM 415 C6415 1985a]
RC495.C533   1990
615.8'512—dc20
DNLM/DLC
for Library of Congress   90-2235
                                                                     CIP

Published by
BRUNNER / MAZEL, INC.
19 Union Square West
New York, New York 10003

Manufactured in the United States of America
10 9 8 7 6 5 4 3 2 1

Contents

Part IV   OTHER CLINICAL APPLICATIONS

Acknowledgments

Many people deserve special recognition for their direct or indirect participation in this book, starting with Virginia Paulsen, the former executive Director of the Colorado Nurses' Association; she always encouraged me to think, explore, and try new things without fear. I miss her and know if she were alive she would be delighted with this undertaking. A supervisor, Dr. H.G. Whittington, first told me that what I was doing was hypnosis and encouraged me to contact my first consultant and teacher, Dr. Wallace LaBaw. He, in turn, encouraged Susan Plock Bromley and me to develop our work with burn patients at Denver General Hospital and supported us through a great deal of self-doubt. But for the opportunity to work with her, I might never have begun practicing hypnosis in earnest. We learned a lot about hypnosis and the processes needed to use it, and those processes were enhanced by working together. Marcia Fishman, who was dragged to one of my workshops by a friend, has gone on to become an expert teacher and clinician in hypnosis. Her contributions to this book are special both in their content and for the fact that, initially, she was not at all interested in the field of hypnosis. Dan Seitzman, Ph.D., supervised me for three years when I was a fellow at the Morton Prince Center for Hypnotherapy; he supported my use of hypnosis with psychotherapy patients to explore intrapsychic processes within a therapeutic relationship.

Dana Schilling, who is not a nurse, read and edited the manuscript in the heat and humidity of a New York summer, trying (I hope successfully) to get me to eliminate as much medical and nursing jargon as possible. Sheila Rouslin Welt, Tricia Berd, Alice Goodloe, Les Muse, Eileen O'Connell, and Dorothy Larkin were all valuable critics. I'm also grateful to Sandy Carrion for typing the rough draft of my chapters. Paul Delany's well-timed story (retold in the conclusion to this book) and intervention motivated me to start writing.

This book is dedicated to the contributors of the book and to my new immediate family: Jay, Jed, Dinah, and to my son Jenda who, now five years older, is called Jonny or Jon. I would also like to recognize Amnon Nadav. I took my first Ericksonian hypnosis course from him several years ago. Amnon died too young in 1989 from a melanoma. As one of his many grateful students and colleagues, I would like to recognize his impact on my development as a hypnotherapist and his subsequent encouragement for and contribution to this book. In addition, I want to thank Norma Ellman for finding all the typos in the 1985 edition.

Preface

Hypnosis and hypnotic techniques are powerful tools for developing and implementing appropriate and effective interventions for myriad health care problems. Long associated with magic, mumbo jumbo, and mysticism, hypnosis has not always been acceptable to the scientific and medical communities. And like the other soft sciences of clinical psychology, sociology, and psychiatry, hypnosis does not always produce consistent, easily generalizable results when scrutinized with the scientific method. Although we still lack clear-cut and consistent explanations about what hypnosis is and how and why it works, more research is produced each year substantiating that an altered state of consciousness can be accomplished and that, as a result of tapping that state, individuals are capable of accomplishing unusual tasks. Such accomplishments might be having major surgery without chemical anesthesia, losing weight, reducing blood loss and blood pressure, recovering completely from a phobia, and visualizing more creative solutions to seemingly insurmountable problems.

Accepted by the Council on Mental Health of the American Medical Association in 1958, hypnosis is now viewed as a valuable tool in medical (health) practice and is used by health caregivers from all disciplines. Today hypnosis is utilized during anesthesia in the operating room as well as during the process of a new-age encounter group. Hypnotic approaches are utilized in many therapeutic schemes ranging from managing stress to stopping smoking to increasing self-confidence and to augmenting the psychotherapy process.

Using hypnosis and hypnotic approaches in evaluating patients and devising interventions is the focus of this book. Originally, when this book was conceived, written, and finally published in 1985, it was directed to a nursing population. However, the book was always intended to be read and used by all health care practitioners in numerous patient care settings. Over the years the book has been used enthusiastically by physicians, social workers, psychologists, physical, occupational, and speech therapists, nutritionists, alcoholism and substance abuse counselors, mental health technicians, psychotherapists, and others who work with people seeking change or repair in their lives.

Compiled by members of several disciplines, the book was, and still is, intended for health care workers in inpatient, outpatient, community, consultation, and educational settings. The first section of the book provides a variety of belief and conceptual systems, theories, and approaches. The second section is filled with clinical case examples drawn from general hospital settings, public health, pediatric, adult, psychiatric, and chemical dependency programs. The identified recipient of care might be an individual, a family member or family unit, a group, a caregiver consultee, or a student. The approaches presented are individualistic; some are considered direct and "traditional," while others are more indirect or derive from the work of Milton Erickson. Many chapters demonstrate a creative integration of theory and approaches that have been clearly designed to meet individual needs.

Clinical Hypnosis and Therapeutic Suggestion in Patient Care is meant to be a theoretical and clinical guide for educators and clinicians. Hypnosis and hypnotic communication can enhance and speed the process of treatment. Although no particular stance or treatise is intended for the work as a whole, it is the editor's belief that hypnosis and hypnotic approaches can be integrated into a total plan of care and are among the many potential therapeutic approaches. Contributing author's preferences for one approach or another are often evident. Authors were encouraged to substantiate their theory and interventions when possible with research and theoretical findings.

The editor also acknowledges that health care is highly complex and most often involves a team approach. When integrating hypnosis into a plan of care, particularly as a direct and named intervention (as opposed to indirect hypnotic communication techniques), the other team members' support needs to be solicited and often they have to be educated about what hypnosis is—and is not. Misconceptions must be dispelled and a unified set of goals and an interdisciplinary team agreement accomplished to potentiate the success of an overall treatment plan.

Although hypnotic techniques are not magic, the results achieved may be dramatic and the process positively engaging for both the client and the practitioner. Hypnosis pulls together the best of health care by combining the art and science of care. Almost limitless in scope and style of approach, hypnosis stimulates the advanced clinician's creativity and challenges the beginner to develop more skills with an easily learned set of interventions.

A SPECIAL NOTE ABOUT THE 1990 EDITION

The editor did not find it necessary to make significant changes in this 1990 edition. Although she acknowledges that more research and writing has been done since 1985, much of the basic theory and conceptual frameworks have remained consistent, and the case examples are timeless in their capacity to teach through example.

When reading chapters where an emphasis seems to be on nursing, the reader need only substitute the word *nurse* with *health caregiver.*

Prologue

This project would have been a more painful experience had it not been for a conversation I had with a co-worker about hypnosis. Paul and I had been sharing stories about how useful hypnotic techniques could be, as we were planning a video taped intervention with one of our patients who had chronic pain and alcoholism. The conversation went from the nuts and bolts of our task to an exciting mingling of ideas about techniques discussed in the book. During this discussion, Paul told me a story, which had a profound effect on me and ultimately on the completion of this book.

When I was a child I had a serious illness, a particularly pernicious form of cancer, which culminated in the loss of my leg at the hip. The whole experience was like a series of shocks. I remember that a trick I used regularly was imagining. Maybe it was just escape, but looking back after more than 20 years, I see that it was a very healthy thing, both physically and mentally. All children fantasize, but I think I recognized that there was a need for me to imagine a better place and a better situation.

I always had specific places I'd go, places I would invent, where I would feel great comfort and ease. Mostly they were natural scenes: a lake in the early morning or a vast green field in a warm sun. Right after I lost my leg, I found it necessary to find a secret place within myself just to get away from the new and awful reality. I had to get away from the doctors and nurses and even my family, because no matter how much support any of them could offer, I knew I was essentially alone with my problem. I would imagine the very early morning at a farmhouse, smoke rising up from the chimney, a scene of utter tranquility. But there was work to be done, and so I would picture the fields and a tractor, cows eating grass next to a fence. This farm was my refuge and my hope at a time when I needed both.

I survived those difficult first days after my amputation, and I like to think I have lived since then, with a certain kind of optimism. In retrospect, I realize that those imaginings were an exercise in survival, an effort to come to terms, by myself, with myself and with a very real world. The farm was a symbol of life for me, a recognition of the need and dignity of work, and a sign that it was time to get up, go out, and tend to my responsibilities. Ironically, I ended up marrying a farmer's daughter, and his farm is really rather like the one of my imaginings.

His story of courage, hope and undaunted determination was very moving to me, both in its content and for his sharing. As the conversation closed I mentioned that I had not been able to begin writing this book. I kept reviewing literature and making outlines of the parts I had to write. I was fearful of starting; it seemed like such an overwhelming task. I had not even unpacked my typewriter. He said, "Get out your typewriter and, when you start, the material will flow. You'll be surprised at how easy it will be; you know the material and what you want to say." That night when I returned home hot and tired from work, I dug out my typewriter and the chapters in this book began. While not always easy, I wrote and wrote often.

This example not only speaks to the importance and potential of hypnotic techniques to Paul but also how useful a well-timed indirect suggestion can be. Paul sought only to encourage me but he managed to say the right thing at the right time and at a moment when I was feeling both awe and wonder at his emotional experience. He told me what I wanted and needed to hear.

This story also demonstrates several points made throughout the book. First, that individuals frequently utilize these techniques on their own, knowing intuitively that they will find relief and new solutions. It is, after all, human nature to imagine and try to find relief from discomfort and tension. Second, seemingly overwhelming conditions can be overcome, and often the first step in that process occurs in the individual's imagination. Third, stories influence human development from childhood until death. Often a message is accepted more clearly through this indirect method than through a more directive approach. Both direct and indirect approaches have been included in the book, and stories are sprinkled throughout to both illustrate a point or to be in and of themselves interventions.

The resources available to those interested in exploring the use of hypnotic techniques continue to grow and are becoming increasingly accessible. Practice and research possibilities seem nearly limitless, and the rewards exceptionally gratifying.

PART I

Conceptual Basis

1

Overview: The Context of Clinical Hypnosis in Health Care*

Rothlyn P. Zahourek

Most health caregivers learn by experience how mind-body processes, suggestion, and the imagination impact illness and recovery. Frequently the patient who says "I won't survive the surgery" dies on the operating table or soon after. The potential for utilizing altered states of consciousness to enhance survival, coping, and recovery, are demonstrated by people who are able to overcome immense odds— for example, a woman completes prepared childbearing without chemical anesthesia; a terminally ill cancer patient disproves a fatal diagnosis and survives; and a burned patient is debrided with little or no pain medications.

Involving individuals actively and positively in their care and helping them to maximize their strengths are goals that most health care providers hold for their patients or clients. Hypnosis and hypnotic techniques are important tools and mechanisms for enhancing people's full participation and for harnessing their greatest potential. Hypnosis and hypnotic interventions also stimulate and challenge the caregiver's creativity to develop individualized approaches.

DEFINITION OF TERMS

Hypnosis

The term hypnosis comes from the Greek work "hypnos," meaning sleep. To date scientists and researchers do not understand the exact nature of hypnosis. Theorists agree, however, that hypnosis is a state somewhere between sleeping and waking, an altered state of consciousness that occurs on a con-

---

*Editors note: Part of the focus of this chapter and some of the examples are related to nursing practice. However, some of the examples could describe caregivers from other disciplines.

3

tinuum of awareness. Hypnosis may occur naturally and spontaneously. Bored in a dull class, our mind wanders, our attention focuses inward, and we become, while still alert and awake, not "there" but rather where our daydream has taken us. When we drive long distances, we often "awaken" with a start, wondering, "How did I get here so fast? I don't remember passing familiar landmarks."

When attention has been keenly focused we may have amnesia, or lack of memory, for the specifics of our daydream. This is a trance state.

Trance

The trance state, often synonymous with the hypnotic state, is characterized by a modified sensorium, an altered psychological state, and characteristically minimal motor functioning. A "wakeful dissociative" state of intense focal awareness, it maximizes involvement with one sensory precept at a time (Spiegel & Spiegel, 1978). Most of us recognize a trance by the individual's glassy-eyed stare, lack of mobility, and nonresponsiveness to external stimuli. A person in a trance state is more receptive to suggestion. In the health care professions, we see patients in naturally occurring trance states. For example, in a waiting room of a busy hospital outpatient department, people sit daydreaming and sometimes dozing in a naturalistic trance state. Too rarely, however, do we consider this an opportune time to give individuals helpful and positive suggestions. In a therapeutic trance state, according to Milton Erickson, the limits "of one's usual frame of reference and beliefs are temporarily altered so one can be receptive to other patterns of association and modes of mental functioning that are more conducive to problem solving" (Erickson & Rossi, 1979, p. 3). Hypnosis, then, is a natural state that can be induced by another or oneself for a specific purpose. It is a therapeutic tool, but not a therapeutic end in itself. As a method of treatment, hypnosis facilitates a number of different treatment modalities (Mott, 1981) and is utilized in conjunction with other approaches to alter psychophysiological states, promote understandings, and allow for creative problem solving.

Suggestion

Webster's New Collegiate Dictionary (1959) defines suggestion as "the mental process by which one thought leads to another especially through the association of ideas" or the "uncritical acceptance of an idea or proposal made by a person to whom the subject is docile and submissive." In the context of hypnosis the dictionary definition is unsatisfactory, perpetuating a myth about hypnosis. In the hypnotic state, the subject is *not necessarily* docile or submissive and may, because of unconscious processes, reject a suggestion given by even the most expert hypnotist.

Kroger and Fezler (1976) described four types of suggestion: (1) verbal, which includes words and any kind of sound; (2) nonverbal, which applies to body language and gestures; (3) intraverbal, which relates to the intonation of words; and (4) extraverbal, which utilizes the implications of words and gestures that facilitate the acceptance of ideas. Suggestions are also described as being direct (obvious) or indirect (metaphor; stories; double binds, and imbedded commands). Suggestibility is a behavior that is uncritically carried out without the individual's logical processes interfering and is enhanced by the client's motivation, expectation, and trust in the operator as well as by the frequency and manner in which a suggestion is given. Additional aspects of suggestion are described in Chapter 3.

Hypnosis Versus Relaxation and Imagery Techniques

The stated goals and procedures differ among these frameworks, (hypnosis, relaxation and imagery) although not markedly. All may evoke an altered state of consciousness and each has the potential for producing a trance-like state. Procedures of induction of the trance state are particularly emphasized in traditional hypnosis and less emphasized in relaxation or imagery techniques. Hypnosis utilizes both relaxation and imagery in the induction procedure, but neither is necessary for the individual to be either suggestible or to enter a trance. Suggestion, which is used in all of the procedures, is most often associated with hypnosis and is utilized consciously and specifically by the therapist. Many also contend that hypnosis purposefully works toward creating a deeper altered state of consciousness where usual superego functions are temporarily suspended. Relaxation, in contrast, focuses on a physiological progressive softening of muscles; imagery utilizes and depends on mental processes; each, however, may be utilized to promote the other.

In practice the differences are more obvious through the patient's (client's) interpretations of the procedures. "Hypnosis" still carries the connotation of magic, loss of control, and being influenced by another or being put "under a spell." Some respond positively to the feelings of "magic" and "mystery," as if something special and powerful is about to be done *to them*. If "suggestive techniques" are mentioned, the patient may interpret the word "suggestion" to mean their symptoms are all of a psychogenic nature and purposely experienced for secondary gain. The power of "imagination" is usually acceptable and carries with it the connotation of something fun, like a game. Relaxation is now commonly accepted by people as a relief for stress and physical and psychological tension. With both imagery and relaxation, the issue of who is doing what to whom and who has the ultimate control seems to be less important than when techniques are labeled "suggestion" or "hypnosis."

The differences among techniques are few and more imagined than real but can enlighten the practitioner when choosing words to use with a client. For example, if a client is anxious about trying hypnosis, use of the term relaxation or imagery might be more acceptable. Regardless of what the technique is called the results may differ little. Although the therapist uses the four techniques somewhat differently, the client experiences all four as similar. The response may or may not be a "trance," however, and variability is to be expected, both among people and within the individual.

Because these techniques are similar, the term "hypnotic techniques" will be applied to relaxation, imagery, and suggestion when all are considered together. The term "hypnosis" will relate to more formalized approaches that utilize suggestion within the context of a purposefully induced trance and may or may not also utilize imagery or relaxation. While hypnosis is the prime focus of this book, "hypnotic techniques" are also described in clinical examples.

ONE HEALTH CARE FRAMEWORK

Recently, educators, clinicians, and scholars across disciplines have sought to develop theoretical frameworks and models to describe a unified mind-body person. Since the 1985 edition, theories have become increasingly biophysiological. Ideodynamic healing, state-dependent learning, and transduction of information are phenomena often described and applied to hypnosis theory.* One useful philosophical framework that can be applied in all disciplines was developed by Martha Rogers, a highly influential nurse-theorist and former nursing dean. She created a model of "synergistic man" (1980). This model describes man as a "dynamic open system" of interactions between and within the self and the environment. A continuum of inner psychic processes affects the individual's relationship to the environment, time, and intra- and interpersonal space. Rogers postulates "phylogenetic and ontogenetic developmental processes characterized by increasing complexity and diversity of pattern organization" (Fitzpatrick, 1980, p. 148). Correlates in this system related to hypnosis include movement from heaviness to lightness to weightlessness; movement from the pragmatic to the imagination to visionary; movement from sleeping to waking to altered states of consciousness.

According to Rogers, because people are whole systems, their behavior cannot be explained or predicted if the components are taken separately. Humans are therefore greater than the sum of their parts. Behavior must be seen as part of a unified whole that cannot be "dichotomized as mental or physical, or as subjective or objective" (Fitzpatrick, Whall, Johnston, & Floyd, 1982, p. 8).

People are dynamic and continuously evolving in complexity and diversity. All aspects of their field—pattern, organization, structure, function, and characteristics—reflect developmental stages and the continuous repatterning of themselves and their relationship to the universe (Fitzpatrick, 1982, p. 8.) Hypnosis and hypnotic techniques are likewise based on these assumptions.

---

*See Rossi (1986) and Rossi and Cheek (1988) in Additional Readings.

the universe (Fitzpatrick, 1982, p. 8). Hypnosis and hypnotic techniques are likewise based on these assumptions.

One last postulate of Rogers related to the subject of this book is, that people by nature are capable of abstraction and imagery, language and thought, and sensation and emotion (Rogers, 1970). This assumption, along with others, has stimulated valuable nursing research and new practice, which have diverged from the classical medical, interpersonal, and/or sociocultural models of care to a more dynamic holistic approach.

One such diversion, fascinating to nurses in recent years and related to hypnotic techniques, has been "therapeutic touch." Krieger, a student of Rogers, developed the "laying on of hands" technique for healing (Krieger, 1979). Krieger emphasized relaxation, imagery, self-awareness, and a therapeutic relationship. A highly personalized interaction develops in which there is ample opportunity for intense emotional involvement from the healer and the healee (therapist and client). As in almost all other relationships, every "psychological ploy" can be acted out to subsequently nullify the positive effects of healing. Transference and countertransference occur because the relationship is open, caring, and nurturing. Because of this, projection, hostility, dependence, passivity, and identification on both parts can occur. Furthermore, because the technique is non-traditional, people seek you out for "nontraditional problems and for which there are no pat answers" (Krieger, 1979, p. 79). Krieger stated that these are often "bêtes noires" (beasts of the night)—creatures unwittingly "fed with the repressed contents of the unconscious and . . . reawakened during illness and increased anxiety" (Krieger, 1979, p. 79). They must not be feared, but rather trusted and utilized therapeutically. The parallel with hypnosis and hypnotic techniques is obvious.

The process of therapeutic touch employs images of color for diagnosis and healing. The healer engages in meditation, which is a "focused, passive act of inattention," and uses relaxation, "centering," and rhythmic breathing. Fast, synchronous EEG activity has characterized the physiology of the healer in this state (Krieger, 1979). This resembles the hypnotic relationship and process. Focused inattention and relaxation aid in receptivity, and vivid imagery intensifies both the healing and hypnotic states. The inherent suggestion in therapeutic touch, that "this is a special and unusual method that will help you and I am going to actively participate in that process with you," again replicates the inherent suggestion in the hypnotic process.

A PARTIAL REVIEW OF THE LITERATURE

In recent years more articles on hypnosis have been appearing in the American nursing literature. Some describe the use of hypnosis with specific cases, while others mention, or describe, the use of relaxation therapy, positive suggestive approaches, or imagery. One of the earliest relevant articles was by

Karen Billars (1970). She never used the word hypnosis in her study on post-operative pain relief. Based on theories of suggestion and the effect of patients' and nurses' expectations, her study evaluated the effect of repositioning and verbal suggestion. Thirty patients recovering from abdominal sugery were divided into three groups, each consisting of ten patients. Group A patients were repositioned and given the suggestion that the intervention would relieve their pain. Group B received the same intervention and suggestion, with the additional reassurance they would be revisited in ten minutes and assisted again if the procedure failed. Group C was repositioned without any verbal suggestion or assurance of additional help. While it was predicted that Group B would have the most pain relief, group A had the most: nine patients had pain reduction. In group B, seven were relieved, and in group C only one had relief. While the sample was small and the study needs replication, Billars speculated that the differences between groups A and B had to do with the strength of the positive suggestion with group A. With group B an element of doubt was interjected when the nurse assured the patient of returning and doing something else if the repositioning did not work. Both groups A and B did much better than group C, which received no verbal suggestions. How often is a procedure done to promote comfort without any discussion of expected results? We might speculate how much more successful ordinary procedures could be with the addition of human contact and positive suggestions.

Bertha Rogers (1972) described therapeutic conversation and posthypnotic suggestion with surgical patients who were stressed and therefore hypersuggestible. She explained how to recognize this state and emphasized the importance of the language and well as the nonverbal communication. "Therapeutic conversation" was used to redirect attention from apprehension, distrust, and discouragement to confidence, trust, and hopeful attitudes. Rogers encouraged the use of imagery, behavioral rehearsal, "cultivating quietness," preoperative suggestion, and recovery room suggestions.

In 1975 an article by Spiegel was published on the myths surrounding hypnosis (Spiegel & Rockey, 1974). In 1977 a classic by Armstrong was published on the altered states of awareness in nursing. Armstrong discussed a theoretical framework for the use of hypnosis and other techniques in which an altered state results. This state is relevant for nursing study in its conceptual scheme of mind and body integration. Nurses are, she emphasized, aware of numerous states of consciousness in their everyday work: awake, asleep, coma, comatose, lethargic, anesthetized, and the "psychopathic and neurotic level found in psychiatry." An *altered state* qualitatively and quantitatively differs from the individual's normally experienced state and is demonstrated by behavior that again differs from one's norm. Armstrong described Benson's (1975) relaxation response, meditation, Simmonton's interventions with cancer patients, and biofeedback as all utilizing an "altered state of awareness." For nursing, these states provide information on the relationship between the body's physiology and mental activities, which are then expressed in behavior (Armstrong, 1977).

Doyle reported a successful hypnotherapy intervention with a case of hysterical blindness. More recent articles have focused on the use of hypnosis by nurse anesthetists (McCoy, 1982), coping with stress (Daley and Greenspun, 1979) (Clark, 1981), obstetrical practice (B. J. Smith, 1982; Vadurro & Butts, 1982), and problem patients who have pain (Zahourek ,1982). Other literature on relaxation and imagery includes Donovan (1981), Sweeney (1978), Achterberg and Lawlis (1982), and McCaffery (1979). Two articles on imagery and visualization in the psychiatric nursing literature report small studies: the first on combating helplessness and the second on developing positive attitudes (Smith, 1982; Vissing & Burke, 1984). A recent book oriented to nursing practice of hypnosis was edited by Boyne (1983). While not scholarly in nature, it provides many practical case examples and descriptions of the hypnotic process used by nurses. *Flynn's Holistic health: The art and science of care* (1980) describes theories of and alternative approaches to promoting wellness and includes practical guides for teaching visualization and relaxation exercises. Likewise, Clark (1981) discussed achieving wellness through numerous routes including imagery and relaxation. Her book has a solid theoretical framework and outlines guides for practically implementing her ideas. Another recent publication on stress, by Brallier (1982), provides relaxation and imagery exercises for nursing practice. These exercises can easily be transposed to the hypnotic relationship.

THE CONTEXT OF CLINICAL HYPNOSIS AND HYPNOTIC TECHNIQUES

Hypnosis and hypnotic techniques are tools used within a larger framework: the therapeutic relationship. Each topic discussed in this book must be viewed within that context. Success seems to be dependent on trust, expectation, belief, and establishing rapport, which exist within that relationship. The following case is drawn from nursing, but the process has application for other disciplines as well.

Choosing a Patient

Except in private practice, caregivers generally do not seek out clients. A caregiver can, however, decide who might benefit from hypnotic or related techniques. Many behavioral scientists are investigating how to choose an intervention based on data obtained from assessment. Some continue to believe that those who do well on hypnotizability scales do best, while others insist that motivation for change makes the difference in outcome. It is generally accepted that the more intelligent, highly motivated patient who expects a positive outcome and is able to concentrate will do the best using hypnosis and hypnotic techniques. An imaginative individual who is willing to trust is also a likely candidate for success. Imbeciles, morons, and maintain focused concentration. Kroger adds that the "scientifically minded may be a poor risk for success because of the inner 'noise' associated with the analysis of emotions" (Kroger, 1977, p. 45). If that scientifically minded person is of a creative or philosophical bent, however, he or she is probably an excellent candidate. (One of the authors' most "hypnotizable" patients was a theoretical mathematician and physicist.) Psychotic, prepsychotic, and severely depressed and suicidal patients should usually also be avoided. Paranoia and delusional thinking can, on occasion, be intensified as a result of the lessening of conscious controls associated with the hypnotic experience.

Therefore, for the beginning practitioner, a motivated intelligent patient who has a specific symptom with little secondary gain is most likely to experience rapid positive results; the caregiver's self-confidence grows and the potential for additional success is augmented. The following nursing example describes the process.

Developing the Relationship

Trust and Rapport

The therapeutic relationship is like making a pot of stew. Before any work can be done, the therapist must establish rapport and trust with the patient. Trust is the meat, the basis for the stew. Trust develops over a period of time and is often tested and retested in relationships. It can, however, be promoted very quickly or be built slowly for therapeutic work.

Hypnosis and hypnotic techniques require some special ingredients. The first is simply getting and maintaining the patient's attention. Another is establishing yourself as a helper and enlisting the patient's cooperation. For example, Mr. Paul has been admitted to the emergency room with abdominal pain. You can establish contact with him by standing in clear view, where eye contact is easily accomplished. You may touch the patient gently, on an unaffected body part if possible, being careful to observe any untoward reaction. Stating your name and position would be the next step. Within a crisis context, the nurse must consider that the patient's attention span and ability to concentrate and remember all might be impaired. Certain sensations are heightened, and hearing becomes selective. Verbal communication must be simple and clear and frequently assessed for patient comprehension. Even in a longer-term relationship, patients are often stressed and anxious when they encounter the nurse. So these steps can apply there as well as when a crisis has developed. Suggestibility is high in both instances.

Establishing rapport is built on initial trust and provides the "sauce for the stew." Without it, the meat will be dry, flavorless, and probably not very successful. Making the sauce requires both direct and indirect procedures. The clinician gains subtle nonverbal understanding by pacing the patient's breathing and mirroring body positions and postures whenever possible. This pacing and mirroring also promotes in the patient a sense that the nurse is in rhythm with him or her. Knowles (1983) discussed several additional techniques from neurolinguistic programming (NLP) theory that build rapport. She described verbal and nonverbal approaches that utilize the person's predominant representational system: visual, auditory, or kinesthetic. People demonstrate their primary mode by such statements as "I *see* what you mean" (visual), "That doesn't *sound* good to me," (auditory), or "I have a *sense* that's a *touchy* issue for you" (kinesthetic). Other senses may also be implied, through statements such as "That *stinks*" or "That leaves a *bad taste* in my mouth." Eye movements and body language also communicate these representational systems.*

While people vary the system during an interaction, most utilize one system predominantly. Because patients under stress regress to their predominant mode and use it almost exclusively, it is important to give information through that mode so it will more likely be remembered (Bandler & Grinder, 1979; Brockopp, 1983). Also, if the nurse is able to pick up how the patient is utilizing information and making decisions and responds with that same system, rapid subtle, empathetic rapport develops. Rapport is also built through feedback of how the nurse perceives the problem or situation. People gain understanding through feedback and feel more in control. Perceptions can be validated or corrected, if inaccurate, and the patient feels the nurse is active and caring.

For example, Mr. Brown is three days postoperative and is sitting upright in bed. He is wide-eyed, picking at the sheets, pale, breathing rapidly, and slightly diaphoretic. The nurse breathes with the patient's rate and rhythm, gradually regulating it as the interaction progresses. Eliminating the possibility of physical problems, the nurse comments while taking his blood pressure, "How are you? You seem worried and tense today. You're fidgeting and don't seem to be able to rest as well as yesterday." He replies, "I'm not worried, but I have more pain today and I can't seem to get relaxed. You all *look* so busy today with all these new people around. I didn't *see* any chance of getting help." He has looked up several times. [Italics are authors.] The nurse replies, "I *see* you are uncomfortable and because we have new students it must *appear* that we are overwhelmed, but we are here to take care of you and it's not as bad here today as it may *look*. Now, let's figure out how we will make you more comfortable."

The nurse does several things in this brief interaction to establish trust and rapport. The patient's obvious behavior is commented on and interpreted. It is reinterpreted correctly by the patient. By monitoring the patient's breathing and noting his nonverbal cues, it is obvious some form of discomfort (tension, worry, pain) is present. Then the nurse utilizes the patient's predominant representational system (visual) and corrects his misperceptions of the environment. The patient is enlisted in the problem-solving process and the nurse

---

*For a complete discussion of NLP theory, see Bandler and Grinder (1979).

positively suggests relief (*not* the absence of pain) will be the result. The nurse also implies, by verbal and nonverbal behavior, a sincere desire to help and a willingness to let the patient know the realities of the milieu. The patient then wants to participate in the process and is motivated to please. This probably enhances the placebo effect of most therapeutic interactions. The patient *expects* positive results.

Motivation and Expectation

Expectation and motivation are the vegetables in the stew. In screening, motivation is partially assessed by evaluating the meaning of the symptoms and estimating the individual's level of emotional stability. Explaining the meaning of certain organic symptoms, dispelling any misconceptions or fears, and communicating expectations of positive results enhance motivation. Expectations are also built through positive direct and indirect suggestions. For motivation to work, the patient must believe in the suggestion as well as in the integrity and well-meaning intentions of the nurse, and most importantly, feel that the ideas given "echo in a profound way the patient's own deeper inner voice" (Crasilneck & Hall, 1975, p. 43).

Returning to Mr. Brown, the nurse tells him directly that it is typical to experience a bit more discomfort on this particular day and that soon he will feel much better. Less directly, the nurse might tell him a story of another (mythical or real) patient who experienced the same problem, used a certain technique, and obtained great relief.

Other patients can sometimes help in building expectations. Helen, a burn patient who used hypnotic techniques successfully for dressing changes, skin grafts, and debridement, was often enlisted to tell other patients how helpful hypnosis had been for her, both for anesthesia and pain management. This not only encouraged others and was living proof that the techniques could have dramatic results but also was a special reinforcement to Helen. She felt like a "star" and was more than happy to share her new sense of mastery with others. Although she was badly burned and occasionally depressed, Helen's positive experience and ability to help others aided her self-esteem (seriously lacking before), thereby further promoting her recovery.

According to Crasilneck and Hall (1975), "Motivation is more than persistence, greater than mere involvement of time in problem solving. It is an emerging process, one whose momentum carries forward in spite of momentary reverses or discouragements. True motivation often pushes relentlessly toward its goal in spite of consciously held resistance. Motivation is the inclusion of hope" (p. 43).

Evaluating and Preparing the Patient for the Intervention

The 'stew' is almost ready, but the cook must choose the right blend of spices to make it delicious. The caregiver in the clinical situation completes the evaluation and decides on an intervention, thus "seasoning the stew."

Evaluating the patient for the use of hypnosis can be a useful part of the therapeutic process itself. This process replicates the nursing process in asking Who, What, Why, and When (defining the problem), choosing an intervention based on the problem, intervening, and subsequently evaluating the results which completes the process.

Crasilneck and Hall (1975, p. 37–39) outlined several questions they ask a patient in *screening* for hypnosis.

1.   Why does the patient come for treatment at this time?
2.   Did the patient decide on treatment or did someone send him or her?
3.   Is the patient motivated sufficiently to give up the symptom?
4.   Does the symptom manipulate others?
5.   Is the symptom organic or psychogenic?
6.   What is the patient's frustration tolerance and ability to control impulsivity?
7.   What is the patient's general personality and history?

This assessment process will, of course, vary if the patient's situation is of an acute or chronic nature. For example, Mr. Paul, seen in an emergency room with abdominal pain, is there for relief of pain. Because of the acute discomfort, he probably agreed with whoever recommended the treatment. He is most likely willing to give up the symptom. He has not had it long enough to use it manipulatively with others. Impulse control may not be an issue, but if he has waited a long time in the emergency room, his frustration tolerance may well be at an end. Whatever is known about the patient can be useful. Is he worried about the cause of pain or does he suspect relatively benign gallstones? What would surgery mean to him at this time? How debilitating will the illness be? Has he tried methods of relaxation or found distraction useful when experiencing other incidents of pain or distress? What else has helped in similar situations?

The initial assessment will be different for Mr. Smith, who has chronic low back pain that has nearly incapacitated him. His wife is fed up with him and has told him that if he doesn't try hypnosis or a related technique, she will leave him. He has come for treatment because of her threat. Mr. Smith verbally states that he wants to give up his pain, but it is clear he has had his family in an uproar, has been on workman's compensation, and expects to stay on disability from a job he never liked anyway. The symptom has an organic base, but everyone who has evaluated him feels that a strong emotional overlay exists. He, furthermore, is known to have a very violent temper and to be generally impatient. One would predict that the intervention with Mr. Smith would entail a longer time and a far more complex process than that with Mr. Paul. Hypnosis or hypnotic techniques could be an appropriate intervention with both cases, but treatment would proceed in a different manner.

To conclude the assessment, and before relaxation, imagery or hypnosis is utilized, the caregiver needs to learn from the patient: What have you done in the past that has helped? What has made things worse? What do you know about relaxation, hypnosis, or imagery? Next, what myths or fears about the chosen hypnotic procedure concern you? Emphasizing that the procedures are safe, and pleasant, and within the patient's control, increases the likelihood of success.

The Intervention

To demonstrate the intervention process, let us examine three examples.

1. Mr. Paul (acute pain, emergency room): Because he has to wait to be seen and diagnosis is pending, no medication has been ordered. He is restless and uncomfortable. The nurse helps him to a more comfortable position and explains why no medication can be given. A brief focused physical relaxation exercise might be chosen. Because time is short, the nurse asks Mr. Paul to focus his attention on one hand and breathe slowly. Suggesting that his hand muscles become limp and that softness, or tingling or coolness might be experienced in the hand diverts attention away from the abdomen. Again the nurse encourages a sense of control, patience, and confidence. If the pain is no longer important diagnostically, glove anesthesia (see also Chapter 9) could be induced and transferred to the abdomen. Suggesting that any sensations indicating an important change would be experienced and reported to the caregivers is often important for continued evaluation.

2. Mr. Brown (three days postoperative): He likes watching television and states that his favorite TV experience was the PBS Henry VIII series. The nurse asks if he would like to promote comfort by visiting that time in his imagination. "As the nurse prepares to give Mr. Brown pain medication she or he could say, "As I give you your medication take some nice breaths and close your eyes. As you relax, the medication will work more quickly. Now take yourself to Henry's court. See the elaborate ballroom with the shining floor, glittering candles, elegant tapestries; hear the wonderful dance music. Smell the fragrant smoke from a blazing fireplace." If the nurse chooses, the patient can, through ideomotor signaling (raising a specific finger to indicate 'yes' or 'no'), communicate if he could see the court and hear the music. The nurse then can tell him that he could dance or simply watch; "whatever you decide you will feel relaxed and comfortable." If Mr. Brown is allowed solid food but has a poor appetite, he might be asked to envision a beautiful banquet. "The table has many of your favorite foods. Taste one of those favorite foods and thoroughly enjoy it." If Mr. Brown appears more relaxed and comfortable, the nurse might then suggest he take a nice nap, awakening feeling refreshed and more comfortable. If he is still restless and uncomfortable, the nurse might continue painting a picture of Henry VIII's court; Henry can even do humorous things—the limits of the scene are dependent only on the nurse's and patient's imaginations.

3. Mr. Smith (chronic back pain):   Mr. Smith's case is longer term. The nurse explains the use of hypnosis or related technique, and that the symptom of pain is so chronic that it has a specific meaning, although that meaning might not be consciously known. If hypnosis is utilized, the patient's unconscious motivation can be explored. For example, the nurse can ask him to become aware of how much pain he needs and how much comfort might make his life better. Using inner dialogue (also see Chapter 5), the nurse might ask the part of his personality that needs the pain to talk to the part that wants to be comfortable. Both parts can express their needs and what purpose they serve. The nurse explains, with the patient in a deeply relaxed state, that both sides can dialogue and gain greater understanding.

The interventions in each of these cases are only suggested techniques. Many are available; the assessment of the patient and the individual nurse's experience, training, and self-confidence will determine the approach taken.

Evaluating the Procedure

It's time to taste the stew. Both nurse and patient are active in evaluating the effectiveness of the technique. Whether it was successful or not, much can be learned both about the patient and about new interventions that might be tried. Because of the vast literature on techniques, many are available for the practitioner to try. Asking the patient, "What did you experience?" and "How did you feel?" aids in the planning of further interventions. If, for example, imagery was tried with Mr. Brown and he stated that his mind kept wandering, the nurse might comment that, while his mind may have wandered, he now looked more relaxed, less diaphoretic, and more comfortable. The patient will probably agree. The nurse might explore where his mind wandered or simply encourage him to relax a specified body part such as a hand to focus attention. As much as possible the patient's experience should be interpreted positively, as that increases the sense of success and motivation to continue. Often practice increases positive results.

In any of the examples, "deepening techniques" might have been tried. These include counting backwards from twenty to one and suggesting that at each number the patient becomes more relaxed and comfortable. Monotonous repetitive phrases and silence can also be used as well as suggestions of increasing relaxation and comfort.

Self-Hypnosis

Because the nurse is not always available, the patient's independent control of symptoms is essential. In teaching patients how to use the techniques, the nurse reinforces self-control and emphasizes that the techniques are not hard to learn, but, like any other skill, need practice for proficiency to develop. Increased independence and the freedom to do the procedure any place or time is stressed to the patient.

The process of teaching the patient is quite standard in the literature on hypnosis and hypnotic techniques. Self-techniques are taught once the patient's cooperation is elicited and he or she has had a positive experience. The following guidelines and instructions for teaching can be used as is or modified to apply in different situations:

1. Be in a comfortable place and position.
2. Say nothing aloud; think the process and the suggestions.
3. Close your eyes and use a key word associated with this state. (This may be a Greek letter as 'delta' or 'sigma' or something like 'relax,' 'peace' or 'calm.' It should be a word to which the patient understands he or she will *only* react with an altered state when that state is desired. Because patients become conditioned to the word, an infrequently used word is often better, although not essential.
4. Take several deep, relaxing breaths and allow your shoulder muscles to relax and your arms to drop and feel heavier.
5. Repeat phrases to yourself such as, "I am getting more relaxed and comfortable."
6. If a scene is visualized, enter that scene as fully as possible, allowing all the senses to be activated.
7. Phrase suggestions positively, for example, "I am getting stronger and stronger" or "I am more and more capable of solving problems, feeling calm, or developing more healthy life styles."
8. If deepening techniques are desired, try counting backwards from 20 or 50 to 1, or imagine yourself going down in an elevator; each floor that is passed promotes more relaxation.
9. Depending on your situation, you might want to suggest a time limit for the procedure, that natural sleep will follow, or that when you count slowly to 3 you will reorient feeling refreshed and invigorated.

It helps to have the patient practice soon after the procedure. Because the experience is fresh and positive, learning takes place more quickly. In the early stages, the patient should avoid any tests of depth, trying to produce any unusual phenomena, or worrying about the depth of the state, since depth is not always related to effectiveness. Commonly, patients report greater depth when the altered state is induced by another. This may be modified with practice and when the patient discovers his/her capacity to promote and enjoy varying degrees of depth. If the patient has difficulty with self-techniques or desires more contact with the clinician than is possible, a tape recording might be made of the specific induction. Standard relaxation, visualization, and self-hypnosis tapes are widely available and can be helpful. Tailor-made inductions, however, are the author's preference.

Teaching Others Hypnotic Technique

Particularly in a general hospital or home situation, family members, significant others, and other staff can all become involved with the patient. Commonly these techniques are tried after a patient has become "problematic." Unrelieved pain, demanding behavior, withdrawal, or intense anxiety leave family members and staff in a quandary about what to do. Due to feeling helpless, these people may avoid the patient, thinking that nothing more can be done. The patient's difficulty only worsens.

These individuals can be informed of the scientific basis of hypnotic techniques. Explaining that relaxation and distraction relieve distress is easily and gratefully accepted by most. If progressive relaxation is used, demonstrating the technique and then emphasizing that the body itself provides the framework encourages people to try the technique. When imagery is to be used, explain that a clearly painted picture helps the vividness of the imagination and promotes greater distraction. Reinforcing key words, and using a monotone, repetition, and silence can increase the depth of the experience and reassures the new helper that the technique is not difficult. Significant others should be cautioned to phrase their comments in a positive way and to *not* add new suggestions. One would not want a family member, for example, removing all pain when the pain was needed for diagnostic purposes or when that pain provides valued secondary gain to the patient. In the same vein, they should be told to immediately report any unusual signs or symptoms before or after using these techniques.

Enlisting the help of others accomplishes not only relief for the busy nurse but also increases the patient's involvement with others. Everyone involved experiences a sense that something is being done and that they have a valuable contribution to make. Feelings of isolation and frustration generally diminish markedly.

PRECAUTIONS

Controversy exists among the experts, but most stress that hypnosis and hypnotic techniques are safe. Considering the number of lay hypnotists practicing on stage and in "hypnosis" clinics, it is amazing how seldom one hears of adverse consequences. (The author does not condone hypnosis for entertainment purposes and feels strongly that such practice has been detrimental to the professional acceptance of hypnosis in particular.) Daydreaming is a common experience for all of us and seldom gets us into trouble unless we become pathologically obsessional or focus on negative thoughts exclusively. Hypnosis should be used with caution, and may be contraindicated in people who tend to habitually retreat from reality, who are chronically detached, or who tend toward too much introspection and daydreaming (Cheek & LeCron, 1968). Probably, progressive relaxation and directed imagery could be helpful with such patients, however. Crasilneck and Hall (1975, p. 308) provided a list of potential dangers of hypnosis to the patient *and* the practitioner:

1. Making an illness worse by indiscriminant symptom removal [pain that is a new symptom is a good example]
2. Causing unncecessary age regression
3. Prolonging treatment with passive-hysterical character-disordered patients
4. Masking other illnesses
5. Providing superficial relief
6. Fantasizing seduction
7. Experiencing panic with relief of superego controls
8. Criminal activity

The authors stressed that all these dangers are eliminated or minimized by proper screening of patients and the use of hypnosis by trained clinicians who are cognizant of psychodynamics. Additional dangers, to the clinician cited by Crasilneck and Hall include (1) excessive grandiosity about the potential of hypnosis; (2) narrowing one's practice to the use of hypnosis exclusively; (3) psychopathological disturbances, e.g., an amateur hypnotist became obsessed with supposed telepathic experiences; and (4) having unrealistic expectations. These dangers are similar to the dangers faced by other clinicians, particularly psychotherapists. They accompany any psychotherapeutic relationship and are most often understood as transference-countertransference reactions.

In summary, caregivers are not to use hypnosis and/or hypnotic techniques indiscriminately with all patients. They should remember that they are valuable tools used within a therapeutic relationship and with a clear understanding of the patient's problem and coping capacities. Hypnosis itself is not dangerous but can be misused if the needs of the patient are not considered (Cheek & LeCron, 1968).

REFERENCES

Acterberg, J., & Lawlis, F. (1982). Imagery and health care. *Topics in Clinical Nursing,* 3, 55–60.

Armstrong, M. (1977). Use of altered states of awareness in nursing practice. *AORN Journal, 25,* 49–53.

Bandler, R., & Grinder, J. (1979). *Frogs into princes.* Moab, Utah: Real People Press.

Benson, H. (1975). *The relaxation response.* New York: William Morrow.

Billars, K. (1970). You have pain? I think this will help. *American Journal of Nursing, 70,* 21–23.

Boyne, G. (1982). *Hypnosis: A new tool in nursing practice.* Glendale, Cal: Westwood Publishers.

Brallier, L. (1982). *Transition and transformation: Successfully managing stress*. Los Altos, Cal: National Nursing Review.

Brokopp, D.Y. (1983). What is NLP?. *American Journal of Nursing, 82,* 1012–1014.

Cheek, D.B., & LeCron, L.M. (1968). *Clinical hypnotherapy.* New York: Grune & Stratton.

Clark, C.C. (1981). *Enhancing wellness: A guide for self-care.* New York: Springer.

Crasilneck, H.B., & Hall, J.A. (1975). *Clinical hypnosis: Principles and applications.* New York: Grune & Stratton.

Daley, T.J., & Greenspun, E.L. (1979). *Stress management through hypnosis. Topics in Clinical Nursing,* 1979, *1,* 59–65.

Donovan, M. (1981). Study of the impact of relaxation with guided imagery on stress among cancer nurses. *Cancer Nursing, 4,* 121–126.

Doyle, D.L. (1977). A case study in hypnotherapy. *American Journal of Nursing, 77,* 806–807.

Erickson, M., & Rossi, E.L. (1979). *Hypnotherapy: An exploratory casebook.* New York: Irvington.

Fitzpatrick, J.J. (1980). Patients' perception of time: Current research. *International Nursing Review, 27,* 148–153.

Fitzpatrick, J.J., Whall, A., Johnston, R., & Floyd, J. (1982). *Nursing models and their psychiatric mental health applications.* Bowie, Maryland: Robert J. Brady.

Flynn, P.A.R. (1980). *Holistic health: The art and science of care.* Bowie, Maryland: Robert J. Brady.

Jacobsen, E. (1929). *Progressive relaxation: a physiological and clinical investigation of muscular states and their significance in psychology and medical practice.* Chicago: University of Chicago Press.

Jacobsen, E. (1967). *Tension in medicine.* Springfield, Ill: Charles C. Thomas.

Knowles, R.D. (1983). Building rapport through neurolinguistic programming. *American Journal of Nursing, 82,* 1011–1014.

Krieger, D. (1979). *Therapeutic touch: How to use your hands to help or to heal.* Englewood Cliffs, New Jersey: Prentice Hall.

Kroger, W.S. (1977). *Clinical and experimental hypnosis* (2nd Ed). Philadelphia: J.B. Lippincott.

Kroger, W.S. & Fezler, W.D. (1976) *Hypnosis and behavior modification: Imagery conditioning.* Philadephia: J.B. Lippincott.

McCaffery, M. (1979). Nursing management of the patient with pain. (2nd Ed). Philadelphia: J.B. Lippincott.

McCoy, L. (1974). Hypnosis—its relationship to anesthesia. *AANA Journal, 42,* 227–232, 1974.

McCoy, L. (1982). Hypnoanesthesia for office surgery. *AANA Journal, 50,* 167–168.

Mott, T. (1981). Hypnosis and phobic disorders. *Psychiatric Annals, 11,* 36–45.

Rogers, B. (1972). Therapeutic conversation and posthypnotic suggestion. *American Journal of Nursing, 72,* 714–717.

Rogers, M.E. (1970). *An introduction to the theoretical basis of nursing.* Philadelphia: F.A. Davis.

Rogers, M.E. (1980). Nursing: A science of unitary man. In Riehl, J., Roy C. (Eds.), *Conceptual models for nursing practice* (2nd Ed.), New York: Appleton-Century-Crofts.

Smith, B.J. (1982). Management of the patient with hyperemesis gravidarum in family therapy with hypnotherapy as an adjunct. *Journal of New York State Nursing Association, 13,* 17–26.

Smith, D.M.Y. (1982). Guided imagination as an intervention in hopelessness. *Journal of Psychosocial Nursing and Mental Health Services, 20,* 29–32.

Spiegel, H., & Rockey, E. (1974). Hypnosis in surgery: exploding the myths. *Surgical Team 3,* 31–37. (Reprinted in *Nursing Digest,* March-April, 1975).

Spiegel, H. & Spiegel, D. (1978). Trance and treatment. New York: Basic Books, pp. 22–23.

Sweeney, S.S. (1978). Relaxation. In Carlson, C., & Blackwell. B. (Eds.), *Behavioral Concepts and Nursing Interventions* (2nd Ed.). Philadelphia: J.B. Lippincott.

Vadurre, J.F., & Butts, P.A. (1982). Reducing the anxiety and pain of childbirth through hypnosis. *American Journal of Nursing, 82,* 620–623.

Vissing, Y. & Burke, M. (1984). Visualization: Techniques for health care workers. *Journal of Psychosocial Nursing and Mental Health Services, 22,* 29–32.

Zahourek, R.P. (1983). Hypnosis in nursing practice: Emphasis on the patient who has pain (parts I and II). *Journal of Psychosocial Nursing and Mental Health Services. 20,* 13–17, and 21–24.

2

Hypnosis: History, Theory, and Controversies*

Maureen Shawn Kennedy
Dorothy Marie Larkin

One new to the concept of hypnosis will find a mind-boggling variety of descriptions, measurement scales, induction techniques, and proclamations as to its nature. Given the very nature of the subject, however, and the inherent problems of conducting research with human subjects, empirical and definitive research on hypnosis has been limited. There are, therefore, several popular viewpoints as to what hypnosis is, who can use it successfully, and what its limitations are.

Rather than provide a laboriously detailed listing of all the contemporary views on the topic, the authors will present two commonly accepted views, chosen largely on the basis of personal preference and familiarity with the respective frameworks. The conceptual discussions will be drawn largely from the work done by Milton Erickson (known for his indirect suggestion techniques) and Herbert Spiegel (known for his development of the Hypnotic Induction Profile and for investigating the correlation between "eyeroll" and hypnotic ability). A brief summation of Kroger's and Hilgard's view are also presented, as they are leading figures in modern hypnosis.

Prior to discussing the works of these modern investigators, a brief review of the roots and history of hypnosis will be helpful in understanding and correcting some myths that continue to plague hypnosis.

---

*The sections on history, controversial issues, and the review of Spiegel's, Kroger's and Hilgard's work were done by Ms. Kennedy, while the sections on the Ericksonian approach and susceptibility scales were done by Ms. Larkin.

HYPNOSIS: A BRIEF HISTORY OF ITS ORIGINS

The earliest roots of hypnosis are found in ancient writings of the Egyptians and Hindus, where rhythmic chanting and drumming was often followed by "temple sleep" or "sacred sleep." It was not uncommon for the believers to experience "visions," "hear voices," or exhibit unusual physiological endurance, such as lying on a bed of nails or walking across hot coals. (On an interesting note, the three prominent Eighteenth Century investigators—Braid, Esdaile, and Elliotson, whose contributions will be discussed below—had all studied or practiced in India.)

It is Franz Anton Mesmer (1734–1815), however, who is credited with being the Founding Father of Hypnosis, although the term *hypnotism* was not used until much later. Mesmer developed what came to be known as the "theory of animal magnetism": he believed the planets influenced humans via a magnetic force, which was responsible for the state of one's health. By applying magnets to the suffering subjects, Mesmer believed he could redirect the magnetic flow and restore health. After a time, he abandoned magnets and used his own hand in a series of "mesmeric passes" over the subject, believing the strength of his own "animal magnetism" could effect cures. His cures were often preceded by convulsions ("crises") and accompanied by the subject experiencing a somnabulistic state.

His clinics in Vienna and in Paris became very popular. To "take the cure," one would sit at "Mesmer's baquet"—a large wooden tub filled with iron particles and water, through which the magnetic force would flow. In 1784, a commission appointed by the French government (one of the members was American statesman Benjamin Franklin) branded him a fraud and denounced his theory of animal magnetism. It is important to note, however, that Mesmer discovered two important factors about hypnosis: the *personal influence* of the operator on the subject's experience, and the achievement of *somnambulism* (walking while sleeping).

A pupil of Mesmer, de Puységur, believed that magnetization induced the somnambulistic state of unusual responsiveness, though he emphasized the will of the operator in controlling the subject (a misconception that persists today).

In 1843, James Braid (1795–1860), a Scottish surgeon, published a treatise, "Neurhypnology (Rationale of Nervous Sleep), in which the term *hypnosis* was first introduced. Braid demonstrated that one could initiate a self-induced sleep by staring fixedly at a bright object (monoidism). He is an important historical figure as he proved mesmeric influence to be personal and subjective. He emphasized that no special power or force passes from the operator to the subject; rather, it is the abnormal suggestibility of the subject to the operator that results in hypnotic phenomena. For the first time, hypnosis was effectively separated from magnetism. The term *mesmerism*, however, persisted in describing hypnotic findings.

John Elliotson was a prominent English physician at the University College Hospital in London, and President of the Royal Medical Society when Braid published his findings. Elliotson followed with his own investigations, and in 1843 published "Numerous Cases of Surgical Operations Without Pain in a Mesmeric State." This paper generated such controversy among his conservative colleagues that he was forced to resign his posts.

It was not until James Esdaile, another Scotsman, presented his data on hypno-anesthesia during surgery that hypnosis became more acceptable as a subject for scientific inquiry. Like Braid and Elliotson, Esdaile had spent time in the Indian Health Service and observed the Hindus' remarkable capacity for somnambulism. Between 1845 and 1847, Esdaile performed surgery using only hypnosis for anesthesia. He published his impressive record (261 operative procedures with a mortality of 5.5%) in 1846 in *Mesmerism in India*.

Braid's ideas on the hypersuggestibility component of hypnosis were championed by two "schools" in France: in Paris by Jean Marie Charcot, and in Nancy by Ambroise Liebeault and Hippolyte Bernheim. Charcot (1825–1893) was a famous neurologist at the Salpetriere clinic in Paris. He saw similarities between Braid's work and his own study of hysteria, which he believed was a psychosis influenced by a patient's ability to respond to suggestion. He viewed hypnosis as a pathological problem similar to hysteria, and in his frame of reference only hysterics were hypnotizable.

While Charcot was using hypnosis to treat hysteria, a former pupil of his, Bernheim, joined with Liebeault in Nancy to study and practice hypnosis. They used hypnotic suggestibility to treat organic illness as well as hysteria. Janet combined the approaches of both the Paris and Nancy schools: he viewed suggestibility as a result of dissociation that can occur in normal mental processes. The work of these early French hypnotists in the 1860s laid the foundation for the discovery and treatment of the neuroses, especially hysteria.

Sigmund Freud, a neurologist, studied first with Charcot and then with Liebeault and Bernheim. He and Josef Breuer used hypnosis as a means of uncovering one's innermost thoughts. Freud was the first to show that dissociated material hidden in one's "unconscious" can later cause dysfunction. (This was the basis for his theory of the unconscious.) He used hypnosis to uncover and revive the original experiences and then to discharge the emotions they had aroused. Later, Freud was to abandon hypnosis for the "free association" technique he made famous.

Although proven successful in the early 1800s for surgical anesthesia and used by reputable and established practitioners such as Charcot, hypnosis never became totally accepted by conservative professionals or the lay public. During World War II, interest in hypnosis was regenerated by the need for short-term therapy (it was often applied in cases of "battle fatigue" or "battlefield neurosis"), and by the combination of hypnosis with more traditional analytic approaches. Mind control and "brainwashing" techniques that came to light during the Korean War again sparked interest in the power of suggestion, especially when the subject is under duress. In the late 1960s and early 1970s, public interest in alternative forms of mental health (transcendental meditation, biofeedback, yoga, etc.) and ways to cope with the stress of the modern world refueled interest in the study of hypnosis.

The nature of hypnosis is still largely unexplained—how it works and why it works better in some than others is yet to be explained or understood, although a variety of explanations have been offered (Perry, Gelfard, & Marcovitch, 1979; Hilgard, 1977; Kroger & Fezler, 1976). The following sections discuss the concept of hypnosis as viewed/practiced by some contemporary figures.

THE PHENOMENON OF HYPNOSIS:
SPIEGEL'S FRAMEWORK

Herbert Spiegel of Columbia University, a leading figure in modern hypnosis, developed the hypnotic induction profile (see also p. 37). This test provides a simple and easily administered test of one's capabilities for hypnosis. While there are varying definitions and descriptions offered about the nature of hypnosis, Spiegel differentiated between hypnosis and other states of awareness (based upon intention and active initiation of the phenomena) as follows:

> Hypnosis is an altered state of awareness in which the individual withdraws his peripheral awareness and concentrates all attention on a focal goal . . . is related to the ability to concentrate in an attentive, responsive manner, even to the point of dissociation. (H. Spiegel, 1972, p. 27)

Spiegel believes that the capacity for hypnosis is innate but that environmental factors can influence this capacity and prevent or reduce one's ability to make use of this phenomenon in a therapeutic manner. Approximately 75 percent of the population has the ability to attain a trance state, with 10 percent being highly hypnotizable (H. Spiegel, 1972).

The Eyeroll Correlation

Spiegel researched large populations and concluded that there is a significant correlation between eyeroll (the amount of sclera visible between the lower eyelid and iris on gazing upward) and the ability to be hypnotized: the higher the eyeroll (Figure 2-1), the greater the hypnotic capabilities. While Spiegel noted this correlation in about 75 percent of the cases (H. Spiegel, 1972), subsequent statistical research has not supported this figure (Hilgard, 1982). Statistical evidence has varied with the populations studied, ranging from no correlation to a high of .52 (D. Spiegel et al., 1982). While actual statistical correlations are disputed, Spiegel believes that (1) a positive relationship between eyeroll and hypnotizability does seem to exist; (2) the eyeroll test can offer a clue to easy identification of hypnotizable subjects; and (3) the

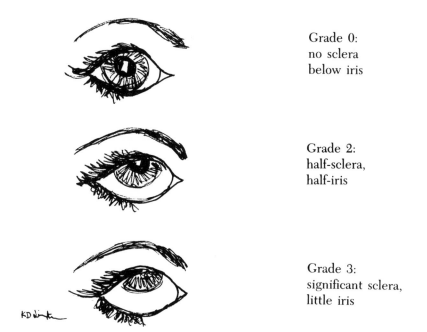

Grade 0:
no sclera
below iris

Grade 2:
half-sclera,
half-iris

Grade 3:
significant sclera,
little iris

Figure 2–1. The Eyeroll is graded according to the amount of sclera visible between the iris and the lower lid when the eye is rolled upward. In grade 4 no iris is visible—only the sclera is seen.

eyeroll may relate to or be a factor of a neurophysiological mechanism that triggers entrance into a trance state (H. Spiegel, 1972). Undoubtedly, there will be considerable research done in this area by supporters and detractors alike. It should be noted that due to individual motivation, even patients with low eyeroll scores can have positive responses to hypnotic intervention. (The scoring of the eyeroll is discussed later in this chapter, under Susceptibility Scales," p. 37.)

Hypnotizability and Personality Characteristics

Spiegel also postulated a relationship between hypnotizability and certain personality traits or "structural themes" (H. Spiegel, D. Spiegel, 1978). He has found that there is a grouping of traits in the lows and the highs that are extremes of each other. In the mid-range of hypnotizability, both groups are represented. Those on the low scale of hypnotizability (grades 0–2) may have a greater need for control in relationships, possess an exaggerated sense of responsibility, a cognitive/analytical approach, and a wider field of concentration. Spiegel termed this group *Apollonian*, though one will recognize the strong resemblance to the traditional label obsessive. Those in the high range of hypnotizability (grades 4–5) tend to be more free-floating, externally influenced (external locus of control), less in need of controlling their relationship, affective as opposed to analytical, and having a more focal or narrowed field of concentration. This group, which he termed Dionysian, corresponds to the traditional *hysteric* label. Some consider it logical that someone with a great ability to be hypnotized (and therefore a great capacity to be responsive to suggestion) would be less controlling by nature, and less analytical and critical.

The Dionysian group comprises only about 10 percent of the hypnotizable population, and experiences very deep trance states—complete somnambulism as well as auditory and visual hallucinations. The grade 5 person can also experience age regression in the present tense, sustain bizarre posthypnotic motor alterations and hallucinatory responses on cue, and has global amnesia of the hypnotic trance state (H. Spiegel, 1974). It is therefore important for grade 5 persons to be identified as highly hypnotizable subjects prior to the choice of treatment modality: because of their hypersuggestibility, traditional analytical therapies can precipitate more confusion and distress, as they explore multiple explanations of a situation. The grade 5 individual will tend to accept suggestions or explanations fairly easily without intense clarification, especially if the explanation is offered by an authority figure. More practical and pragmatic approaches are suggested for these individuals (H. Spiegel, 1974).

MYTHS VERSUS FACTS ABOUT HYPNOSIS

There are several popular misconceptions about hypnosis, and the clinician planning to employ hypnosis in practice will often have to educate the client before he or she will accept hypnosis as a bona fide treatment or assessment adjunct. The major myths and a discussion of each follows.

Hypnosis Is Similar to Sleep.   This is perhaps the most perpetuated and most incorrect of all the misconceptions surrounding hypnosis. The word hypnosis is derived from the Greek word *hypnos* (to sleep), but from what is known today of both sleep and hypnotic states, it is safe to say that they are at opposite extremes of the sleeping–waking continuum. Hypnosis is a state of attentive concentration, so much so that peripheral awareness is withdrawn, while focal awareness is heightened to the point of dissociation in some individuals. In sleep, however, *both* peripheral awareness and focal concentration are withdrawn.

Hypnosis Is a Sign of Mental Weakness or Instability.   Hypnosis has been identified as a state of altered attention requiring increased and sustained concentration. Pathology that interferes with concentration (such as schizophrenia) makes it nearly impossible for one to be hypnotized. Hypnotizability is more likely to be a sign of mental health than of mental weakness.

The Hypnotist Is In Control of the Subject   The subject consents and chooses to be responsive to the instructions of the hypnotist and thereby has control. The hypnotist merely guides the subject into the trance state. That self-hypnosis is possible at all is evidence that the hypnotist is incidental to the process. In this sense, all hypnosis is actually self-hypnosis. During the therapeutic process, the clinician will make use of the client's heightened concentration and responsiveness to suggestion in treatment strategies. It is, however, extremely important for the therapist to keep in mind the very extreme responsiveness of the Grade 5 individual (see the following paragraph) when suggesting various alternatives, whether or not the patient is in a trance state.

People Cannot Be Made to Do Anything Abnormal or Against Their Normal Beliefs.   Some question exists about whether or not the above is true. The Grade 5 hypnotizable person (high capacity for responsiveness to suggestions, global amnesia following the event, and a tendency to be very trusting and noncritical) is very vulnerable. This type of person tends to be the object of the entertainer-hypnotist demonstration, and can be made to act in ways he or she does not remember or believe when the trance state is ended. The parlor tricks and stage routines are usually not harmful to the subject, who rarely suffers more than embarrassment or anxiety. It should be pointed out, however, that the Grade 5 person will often respond to suggestions or statements *not* intended as actions for that person to carry out (H. Spiegel, 1974), so caution is recommended.

Hypnosis is Dangerous.   Hypnosis is a natural phenonmena, and of itself is not a dangerous thing. Like any ability improperly assessed or used indiscriminately by an unskilled clinician, undesirable results can occur.

Symptom Removal is Dangerous.   It has been believed but not substantiated that the removal of a symptom will give rise to another perhaps more dangerous or disabling symptom. Hypnosis is an effective way to enable clients to achieve mastery and control without prolonged investigation into the origins or meaning of symptoms. However, symptoms do have meaning and may not abate when secondary gain is important. Again, with careful assessment of the client, the importance of the symptom should become clear. With a supportive therapeutic environment that does not force or coerce the client to abandon the symptom and simultaneously allows for retrieval of the symptom if needed, there is no reason to presuppose that symptom removal will create harm or discomfort (H. Spiegel, 1967; Holland, 1967; Kroger, 1977; H. Spiegel & D. Spiegel, 1978).

KROGER'S FRAMEWORK

William Kroger defined hypnosis as a state in which the subject allows the therapist to place restrictions on his or her sensory and cognitive perceptions, and in this state the subject recognizes only those stimuli the therapist permits. It is the patient's selective attention and expectations that allow hypnosis to occur. The interpersonal relationship between the patient and the therapist is an important factor in whether or not hypnosis will be successful.

Like most practitioners, Kroger believes that hypnosis is a natural and frequently occurring phenomenon. It is a magnified or heightened extension of normal attentive awareness. As such, hypnosis is not in itself dangerous; rather, any danger results from improper patient selection or inappropriate use of the technique by the practitioner. Kroger feels that the use of permissive, non-authoritian suggestions according to the needs of the patient allows the letting-go of symptoms by those who can do without the disturbing behavior. Another technique offered by Kroger is the removal of a disturbing symptom coupled with substitution of a less offensive symptom. Kroger disclaims that hypnosis itself can cause psychosis, but he does caution that if a psychotic process is in place, an acute event may be precipitated by hypnosis.

ERNEST HILGARD—"THE HIDDEN OBSERVER"

Hilgard has spent over two decades in hypnotic research, and prior to that, a decade in research on learning. His major contribution and most revealing research has to do with his concept of "the hidden observer"—the hypnotized subject's dissociated processing of events outside awareness while in a hypnotic trance state.

In Hilgard's studies, pain or deafness was experimentally induced in the laboratory setting, and subjects were asked through a hypnotic suggestion to indicate if any part of them experienced pain or could hear. This was done by either raising a hand/finger, or by "automatic writing"—under hypnosis the subject revealed by handwriting that sound or pain was indeed processed. When out of the hypnotized state, the same subject was consciously unaware of having written or of hearing anything or feeling any pain. On a cognitive awareness level, the subject did not experience the stimuli, yet it was processed and experienced on another level. There should be considerable research in this area in the near future.

INTRODUCTION TO THE ERICKSONIAN APPROACH

Any attempt to adequately discuss Milton Erickson's principles and philosophy of hypnosis would require the inclusion of volumes of manuscripts, books, and videotapes. Consequently, the following treatise will only include selected hors d'oeuvres to whet the appetite for the numerous main courses yet to come. In order to more fully understand how much is available to learn, the reader might only need to enjoy experiencing a developing sense of curiosity. This curiosity can inspire the intellect to find appropriate Ericksonian literature which will further enhance the pleasures of curiosity and thereby provoke additional craving for more intellectual satiation. The unconscious can then create a medley of surprises (frequently consciously recognized retrospectively) which will demonstrate just how applicable Ericksonian hypnotic techniques are within the nursing profession.

Erickson's renowned hypnotic capabilities evolved from a fairly nontraditional background. As an adolescent he contracted polio. He later described the affliction as "a terrific advantage over others" (Erickson & Rosen, 1982, p. 47), since the ability to move only his "eyeballs" enabled him to discover the pleasures of astute observation. While quarantined on the family farm in Wisconsin with seven sisters, one brother, two parents, and a practical nurse, he learned the intricacies of nonverbal communication and the frequency of conflicting verbal counterparts. His tone deafness was also an asset; he was "forced to pay attention to inflections in the voice" and was hence "less distracted by the content of what people say" (Haley, 1967, p. 2).

Although informed he would never walk again, Erickson became acutely aware of the nature of progressive movements by watching how his creeping baby sister learned to stand up. He reportedly spent hours concentrating on creating a flicker of movement in his legs, and once he succeeded, he continued by carefully noting and directing the incremental progression of returning mobility. Within a year he was on crutches. The following summer, at the age of 17 and with the strength to swim only a few feet, he took a 1200 mile solo canoe trip (his physician had recommended that he build up his arm muscles). Clearly his personal history manifests his philosophy that patients can and should develop their assets and extend their perceived limitations. This trip also provided Erickson with the opportunity to discover how assistance can be obtained without directly asking for it. Although he was initially too weak to carry his canoe over a dam, he was able to shinny up a nearby pole. He took with him a preparatory medical book, which he began reading while perched on top of the pole. This odd behavior secured a curious group of observers and when someone inevitably asked him what on earth he was doing, Erickson looked up from his book, and replied that he was waiting to get his canoe carried over the dam. The observers were then free to and did volunteer their services.

Erickson obtained an M.D. and an M.A. in psychology and continued his education in hypnosis. His personal capacity to utilize hypnosis for the promotion of comfort and healing was further developed when at the age of 51, he was afflicted with another strain of polio. Although markedly weakened on his right side, within a year and with the assistance of two canes, he completed one of the more difficult hikes in Arizona. For health reasons, he settled in Phoenix, where he developed and maintained an active private practice in his home. He was founder and president of the American Society of Clinical Hypnosis, became the founding editor of the *American Journal of Clinical Hypnosis*, published over 100 papers, and lectured extensively on trance induction, experimentation, and clinical techniques. His death in 1980 enhanced the growing recognition that the work and philosophy of this unique scholar should be preserved and promulgated. The Milton H. Erickson Foundation was established in Phoenix, and this group conducts international Ericksonian conferences and maintains a library of donated video and audio tapes. Books, workshops, and local Ericksonian societies continue to sprout with remarkable resiliency for the benefit of interested professionals.

Ericksonian Concepts

Erickson defined hypnosis as "a communication of ideas and understandings to a patient in such a fashion that he will be most receptive to the presented ideas and thereby motivated to explore his own body potentials for the control of his psychological and physiological responses and behavior" (Erickson & Rossi, 1980, p. 237). He also stated that "in hypnosis what you want your patient to do is to respond to an idea. It is your task, your responsibility, to learn how to address the patient, how to speak to the patient, how to secure his attention, and how to leave him wide open to the acceptance of an idea that fits into the situation" (Erickson & Rossi, 1981, p. 42). He emphasized that the average person is unaware of the extent of his or her capacities and that unrecognized unconscious learnings can be employed and developed with the aid of effective communication. Erickson described the role of the operator as "a source of intelligent guidance," and his experience has been that "the less the operator does and the more he confidently and expectantly allows the subjects to do, the easier and more effectively will the hypnotic state and hypnotic phenomena be elicited in accord with the subject's own capabilities" (Erickson & Rossi, 1880, p. 15). He encouraged users of hypnosis to be fully cognizant of *all* types of hypnotic techniques so that each hypnotic experience can be tailored to fit the individual and the specific situation. He repeatedly emphasized the futility of rigid, standardized techniques because they do not take into account the variability of human behavior.

Although he did not like labels to describe his own approach to therapy, he reluctantly agreed that "eclectic" could be an appropriate description. As defined by the American Heritage Dictionary, this word stems from the Greek word Eklegein, "to single out, choosing or consisting of what appears to be the best from diverse resources" (Moore, 1982).

Erickson's basic impression was that each individual enters every situation with both a conscious and an unconscious mind. Therapeutic communication can be directed to the unconscious, creative, more intelligent part of the mind by interspersing suggestions within the basic, usually more mundane conversation to the conscious mind. The recipient is then free to choose how and when to enact the various appropriate suggestions for creating change.

Erickson's principles are versatile and can be employed in a variety of different therapeutic situations. For example, his well-known hypnotic induction on the process of learning (Erickson, Rossi, & Rossi, 1976) can be individualized to many different clinical problems. One can learn to alter the perception of pain, enjoy losing weight, relax, etc. Success can most often be ensured when the individual perceives the change to be obtainable and uplifting. An effective facilitator needs to offer a rational presentation on how that change can be obtained, although the suggestions might need to be qualified with a comment such as, "Perhaps your unconscious already knows a better way and will demonstrate that to you at the proper time." The subject is then free to direct the creation of that change either via the suggested methods or by something completely different. The facilitator needs to remember it doesn't really matter how a therapeutic change is created as long as the individual perceives it as intrinsically appropriate. Erickson supported Milgram's 1963 premise that no utilization of hypnosis can elicit behavior contrary to the subject's wishes, backgrounds, training, better judgments and even moral sense" (Erickson & Rossi, 1980, p. 16).

Utilization and Confusion Techniques in Health Care

Ericksonian principles are easily incorporated into clinical practice by employing his "utilization technique" (Erickson, 1959). Initially this involves accepting the patient's current behavior and experience. Then, utilizing some part or parts of that experience, the nurse gently redirects the patient's perceptions inwardly and toward a therapeutic goal. For example, a 19-year-old female patient of mine with second- and third- degree burns over 60 percent of her body required frequent daily exercises to prevent the development of muscle contractures. One day as her arm was being painfully flexed, she suddenly screamed, "It's pulsing, I can feel it pulsing!" I accepted and promptly utilized this perception, responding with "Yes, and I wonder if your count of those beats will be the same as my count as I take your pulse." The patient's sudden altered expression indicated absorption with the suggested task, and 15 seconds later we both agreed that the count was 22 beats. I then offered a brief description of the process of biofeedback, explaining how some people can learn to reduce their heartbeat merely by taking a few deep breaths and thinking about it. I then suggested that perhaps the back of her mind would demonstrate to her how that can be done. Further flexion was required for her to perceive those beats (a process that was consistent with my own therapeutic intent), and our agreed count after 15 seconds diminished to 19 beats. Complete flexion was obtained just as her attending occupational therapist arrived and exclaimed with delight, "How did you do that!?" I simply and emphatically replied, "She now knows how to continue to do it." This generalized indirect implication for future success was validated throughout her remaining rehabilitation period. As she continued to associate her exercise period with an opportunity to practice this learned capability, she concomitantly discovered that this process of concentration also increased her sense of comfort and relaxation. She was released from the hospital with full mobility and consequently did not require the expected subsequent operations for contracture release.

The utilization technique is often incorporated within other Ericksonian techniques, and can be recognized in a number of different effective inductions. Erickson reportedly discovered the impact of confusion when a harried young man rounded a corner and collided with him. Before the proper expected apologies could be extended, Erickson calmly looked at his watch, informed the man that it was exactly 10 minutes of 2 (it was actually closer to 4:00), and then strolled away. Noting that the bewildered gentleman appeared to be still disoriented from half a block away, Erickson began to formulate his understandings of the therapeutic potential of confusion (Erickson, 1964). An important characteristic of the confusion technique is that it jolts an individual's attention away from the prevailing situation and then suggestively redirects it toward a more therapeutic goal.

Since the majority of patients expect the health professional to communicate meaningfully and rationally, the therapist who occasionally deviates from this role by offering situationally inappropriate and irrelevant comments is likely to induce a hypnotic trance state. The astute practitioner should be able to observe the patient's sudden alteration of perceptual awareness and can then direct his or her attention by providing appropriate suggestions. If the subject appears to be not attentive to what is being communicated, then the therapist should change some aspect of the intended therapeutic strategy. The patient's attention might be successfully recaptured by either reverting back to the utilization technique or by offering another completely irrelevant and confusing comment.

An example from my nursing practice follows:

I was still on orientation in a pediatric bone marrow transplant unit when three other nurses requested assistance in holding down a thrashing 6-year-old girl (whom I will call Tina), who had recently been diagnosed as having Fanconia's pancytopenia (a rare genetic anemia which had already killed three of her sisters). Although it was time for her daily dressing change, she preferred today not to have anyone touch her wounded and painful leg. The following conversation ensued.

RN: Tina, have you met Dorothy? She's a new nurse here.
D: (Tina looked at me. I moved closer, captured her gaze, focused at eye level, and spoke in a slow and intent deep voice.) Is it all right if I call you Fred?
T: (Tina appeared shocked, paused, seemed to momentarily internally evaluate the unusual implications of such a question, and then in full force shouted) NO!
D: Oh, well, okay . . . How about George?
T: (Another momentary pause, and then, loudly and indignantly) I'm a GIRL!
D: (Again Tina's comment is accepted and utilized.) Yes, well, I'm a girl too, and it's all right if you call me Fred. (The implication here is that it's okay to pretend, and that just because something is unquestionably what it is doesn't mean it can't be made to seem different. It was hoped that this concept could then be generalized to include her experience of pain.)
D: (While Tina was considering this comment, I sat behind her and hugged

her with gentle restraint. The other nurses began to quickly cut away her dressing while I whispered secret challenging questions into her ear.) Bet you don't know how many muscles you use when *you lift that leg*. (Note the direct interspersed suggestion* with use of dissociative phrase that leg.")

T: (In order for Tina to find out how many muscles are needed to lift that leg, she had to lift it, which she did. As she began to demonstrate her counting ability, the other nurses pulled off her dressing. This action evoked another altered thought process, and she responded by squirming and repeatedly screaming . . .) Ouch!

D: (I again accepted and utilized her response by counting the ouches, and then asked Tina if she could jump from four ouches to six ouches without saying five," a confusing intellectual question for a 6-year-old. Adults would probably reject this immediately whereas a child might stop to consider. She hesitated to consider this and appeared to be internally absorbed when I intently whispered a permissive suggestion.) And it can hurt just for the time it takes you to say "ouch."

D: (I continued to hold Tina's attention by asking her questions which both evoked her curiosity and required her own perceptual assessment before she could know the answer. This change in perceptual attention is theorized to close the "sensory gate" to incoming painful stimuli [Melzack & Wall, 1965].) How short can you make your "ouches"? Do you need to push your tongue against your teeth as quick as you can to make a tiny little ouch? (Tina began to experiment with different oral methods of condensing and elongating "ouches." She appeared to experience relatively little pain throughout the rest of the dressing change, since she giggled between each emitted "tiny little ouch.")

Humor can also evoke a sudden change in perceptual awareness, and Erickson's work is replete with examples. Recent indications that laughter may stimulate the immune system and enhance endorphin production imply additional therapeutic benefit for the patient (Cousins, 1979; Moody, 1978).

The former two examples provide only a cursory appreciation of Ericksonian approaches as applied in the nursing profession.* Multilevel communication offers opportunities limited only by the number of situations in which they are applied. The humanistic character exemplified by each Ericksonian encounter illustrates the value of benevolent ethics and holistic care. As techniques evolve into therapeutic art, individual styles will find principles for practice in the many examples of Erickson's judgment and respect for his patients' highest potential.*

---

*See Chapter 3 for further discussion of the use of indirect suggestions.

*More references to Ericksonian approaches can be found in Chapters 3, 11, and 13.

*The author extends appreciation to Joseph Barber Ph.D., Leonard Lewenstein M.D., Kay Thompson D.D.S. and Amnon Nadar M.A. for critical and constructive review of the portions on Ericksonian approaches in nursing.

CONTROVERSIAL ISSUES SURROUNDING HYPNOSIS

Since the very nature of hypnosis makes for difficult empirical research, concrete and absolute verifications about its dynamics are rare. Thus, much of the arguments about its various facets can be substantiated from both points of view. Controversial issues today seem to revolve around clinical measurement (whether there is indeed a neurophysiological factor such as the eyeroll correlation) and the clinical employment of hypnosis for various somatic or behavioral problems.

The question of who should be authorized to use hypnosis professionally is also controversial. Traditional medical hierarchy claims hypnosis belongs in the province of physicians, dentists, psychiatrists, and psychologists; evidence of this is the restricted membership of the Society for Clinical and Experimental Hypnosis. However, there is increasing evidence of study and practice of hypnosis by nurses and social workers within their respective frameworks. The AFL-CIO also has a group of lay (non-health care professional) hypnotists.

What is more important than *who* is using hypnosis is *how* they are using it. If used judiciously by someone adequately trained and within the context of legitimate and ethical goals, there is no reason or inherent right for one group to lay claim to its use.

HYPNOTIC SUSCEPTIBILITY SCALES

One of the major controversies among hypnotherapists relates to susceptibility scales. (These scales, modified for children, are discussed in Chapter 10.) The quest for a standardized scale that can effectively measure an individual's hypnotizability has been subjected to years of scale modifications, revisions, and professional debates. Hypnotizability is perceived by some clinicians as an innate biological capacity (H. Spiegel, 1972), which is expected to be only present in a certain quantifiable portion of the population. Other practitioners maintain that any individual with an ability to focus attention can enjoy the experience of hypnosis. This group argues that the unique intrapsychic circumstances of both the subject and the therapist combined with the prevailing environmental situation can render any standardized technique ineffective. They assert that it is the therapist's responsibility to choose an induction that will conform to the needs of each subject. They also encourage clinicians to be prepared to utilize the opportunities presented by individual variation, so that a hypnotic trance can be secured for the subject who "resists" standardized techniques. This premise has been clearly described by M. Erickson (1952, p. 72):

> When thought is given to the difficulty of "standardizing" such intangibles as
> inter- and intrapersonal relationships, the futility of a rigid hypnotic technique

"to secure controlled results" is apparent. An awareness of the variability of human behavior and the need to meet it should be the basis of all hypnotic techniques.

Cooper and London (1978–79) defined susceptibility as "the frequency [with which] a subject acts as a hypnotized person when the responses are elicited by the standardized procedure" (p. 170). The resultant evaluation is only applicable for that standardized procedure since a defined unsusceptible subject in a particular study might well be highly susceptible to a more individualized approach in another. This important distinction can help clarify the interpretations offered in clinical and experimental hypnotic research.

One early predecessor of hypnotic susceptibility scales was developed by Friedlander and Sarbin (1938). This scale purported to measure a subject's responsiveness to hypnosis by appraising such items as eye closure, catalepsy, posthypnotic hallucination, and posthypnotic amnesia. In 1959 Weitzenhoffer and Hilgard restandardized this form with slight modifications and additions to create the *Stanford Hypnotic Susceptibility Scale, Forms A and B* (SHSS:A and SHSS:B). Correlation with the Friedlander–Sarbin scale was found to be .95 (Hilgard, Weitzenhoffer, & Gough, 1958), and hence they proposed both scales similarly measured typical behaviors and experiences of hypnotized subjects. Later scales have employed these basic scales as a reference for comparison and evaluation of statistic correlations. When the statistical correlation proved high (the maximum correlation is $+1.00$ for a perfect positive relationship; Hilgard, 1978–1979), it was assumed that the newly developed scale was adequate for measuring hypnotic susceptibility. Any inherent limitations in the initial scales might have subsequently been perpetuated in the later scales in an effort to procure maximum correlations. Susceptibility scale skeptics might argue that the prevalent professional disagreement regarding the merit of any standardized scale further supports the premise that they were insufficient at their onset and then just had their insufficiencies further developed.

A few of the common susceptibility scales utilized in hypnotic research are summarized here. The original sources are provided in the References for those interested in a more detailed description of these scales.

The Stanford Hypnotic Susceptibility Scales, Forms A and B (SHSS:A and SHSS:B) consist of 12 items which are scored pass or fail. They begin with a waking suggestion item known as the postural sway. Before the hypnotic induction is offered, the subject is given the suggestion to fall backwards and if necessary be caught by the hypnotist. A compliant response is scored as a pass. This is followed by an induction similar to Friedlander and Sarbin's, which consists of suggested eye closure while viewing a target. If the subject's eyes close, this item is scored as a pass. The remaining 10 items consist of hand lowering, arm immobilization, finger lock, arm rigidity, moving hands, verbal inhibition, hallucination, eye catalepsy, posthypnotic suggestion, and amnesia.

The *Stanford Hypnotic Susceptibility Scale Form C* (SHSS:C) was developed in 1962 by Weitzenhoffer and Hilgard because it was decided that the SHSS:A and SHSS:B evaluated too many motor functions and not enough cognitive distortions. The 12 items are measured on a pass or fail basis. The items include hand lowering, moving hands apart, mosquito hallucination, taste hallucination, arm rigidity, dream, age regression, arm immobilization, anosmia to ammonia, hallucinated voice, negative visual hallucination (seeing two out of three boxes), and amnesia. The reliability of the total Form C score was estimated to be .85, about the same as SHSS:A and SHSS:B.

In 1963 and 1967, the *Stanford Profile Scales of Hypnotic Susceptibility, Forms I and II* were developed by Weitzenhoffer and Hilgard to select subjects for participation in experiments that required special hypnotic talents and to differentiate between moderately highly and very highly hypnotizable subjects. These more diagnostic scales were designed for those with a fair degree of hypnotic talent, and consequently it was suggested that subjects who score 4 or less on SHSS:A be omitted from the testing. To reduce the time requirements of the SPS tests, an alternative "tailored" SHSS:C was developed for the selection of subjects with special hypnotic talents. This scale enables the investigator to replace one item of SHSS:C with a special item considered appropriate for the proposed study (Hilgard, Bowers, Crawford & Kihlstrom, 1977).

Two shorter scales developed for clinical use are the *Stanford Hypnotic Adult Clinical Scale* and the *Children's Hypnotic Clinical Scale* (Morgan & Hilgard, 1979). They are considered to be satisfactorily reliable and capable of providing special information on special hypnotic abilities.

The *Harvard Group Scale of Hypnotic Susceptibility, Form A* (HGSHS:A) was developed by Shor & Orne (1962) and has been adapted from the SHSS:A for group administration and self-scoring. Nine of the 12 test items are considered to be essentially the same as SHSS:A, and the others have been designed to test similar functions. Correlation of observer and self-scores was found to be .83 for group sessions and .89 for individual sessions (Bentler & Hilgard, 1963). The reliability, convenience, and time-saving characteristics of this scale render it a common choice of investigators.

The *Children's Hypnotic Susceptibility Scale* (CHSS) was developed by London in 1963. This scale consists of 22 items, 12 of which were modified from SHSS:A and B; the others were based on the unpublished Stanford Depth Scale (Hilgard, 1965). All items were rewritten to make them more appropriate for use with children. An important new component in this scale was the inclusion of subjective scoring along with the usual objective scoring, and it was reported that the paired results were highly correlated.

The *Barber Suggestibility Scale*, developed by Barber & Glass in 1962, was constructed to test hypnotic-like behaviors in a situation that could either be defined as hypnosis or as a test of the imagination. This scale includes eight standardized test suggestions (arm lowering, arm levitation, hand locking, suggestion of thirst, verbal inhibition, body immobility, posthypnotic suggestion of a cough, and selective amnesia), and asks the subjects to imagine and then experience the suggested effects. Scoring is obtained by both objective and subjective reports. This scale was found to correlate .62 to .78 with the SHSS:A and is considered to be a valid and reliable measure.

In 1978 Wilson and Barber developed the *Creative Imagination Scale* in an effort to reduce the authoritarian tendencies of previous scales. This scale consists of ten permissive test suggestions that "guide subjects to use their own thinking and creative imagining in order to experience the suggested effects" (p. 91). The items are arm heaviness, hand levitation, finger anesthesia, drink-of-water hallucination, olfactory–gustatory hallucination (smelling and tasting an orange), music hallucination, temperature hallucination, time distortion, age regression, and mind-body relaxation. Subjects are administered a self-scoring form which rates their experience on a five-point scale ranging from "not at all the same" (score of 0) to "almost exactly the same" (score of 4). This scale can also be administered to a group.

The *Hypnotic Induction Profile* * *(HIP)* is a simple measurement tool that provides a 5 to 10-minute assessment of a subject's hypnotizability. It consists of an actual induction into a trance state along with measurements of eyeroll, which Spiegel considers a biological indicator of trance capacity and one's ability to be responsive to a series of instructions. The HIP was standardized on 3232 patients in psychotherapy over a 3½ year period. Eyeroll and the HIP are both scored on a numbering system of grades 1 to 5, with 4 and 5 representing high hypnotizability, 2 and 3 representing moderate hypnotizability, and 0 and 1 representing no or little hypnotizability. According to Spiegel, a high eyeroll score can be expected in most cases to be a reliable predictor of hypnotizability. Spiegel claims an individual who demonstrates a high eyeroll score but an *inability* to be hypnotized should be evaluated for the presence of severe psychopathology (H. Spiegel & D. Spiegel, 1978; H. Spiegel, 1974a). This combination of a high eyeroll without other positive substantiating measurements in the HIP constitutes a "decrement" or "soft" profile, indicating a break or total collapse of concentration.

The HIP as a clinical tool can uncover selective information relative to the patient's responsiveness to direct, standardized forms of hypnotic inductions. While a grade 4 indicates responsiveness to direct suggestion, subjects with a grade 1 or 2 who are motivated to change can be successful in employing hypnosis toward that goal (Spiegel & Spiegel, 1978; Shafer & Hernandez, 1978). Subjects not scoring well on the HIP may be more receptive to indirect individualized hypnotic suggestions. More research is needed to clearly systemitize this process. Clinicians skilled in both direct and indirect hypnotic approaches can tailor their techniques to fit the unique needs of each patient.

The *Hypnotic Induction Profile* (H. Spiegel & Bridger, 1970), with its

---

*This tool is controversial, as is the importance of "hypnotizability" in both the study and practice of hypnosis (for a complete description of the HIP see H. Spiegel and D. Spiegel, 1978).

controversial eyeroll sign (Frishholz et al, 1981; Hilgard, 1981; Spiegel, 1972), was described by the investigators as practical because it could be administered in the clinic in five to ten minutes. The brevity of this procedure prompted their recommendation that it be used as a screening measure because "if an individual shows little evidence of clinically usable hypnotic capacity, therapy using hypnosis may not be the method of choice" (Stern, Spiegel, & Nee, 1978–1979, p. 109). Individuals labeled grade 0 or 1 can leave the screening procedure with the implicit professionally suggested belief that he or she is unsusceptible to hypnosis. These subjects will remain skeptical of having any hypnotic capacities unless they receive appropriate education. They should be informed that a low susceptibility score only indicates that the subject was not susceptible to that particular test at that particular time. They should also be made aware that susceptibility scores say nothing about basic capacities nor about ultimate clinical outcome" (Barber, 1980, p. 61).

Cautions Regarding Susceptibility Tests

Skeptical clients tend to quickly comprehend the inherent limitations of susceptibility scales when provided with a brief description of Barber's "sleep susceptibility" analog (Barber, 1980). This refers to a hypothetical study in which a fully rested individual is escorted into an experimental environment of relaxation and comfort. Lullabies, soft music, calming colors, and a bedtime story further enhance the nocturnal ambiance. The subject lies down on a perfectly comfortable bed, and if sleep does not occur within the predesignated 15 minutes, he or she is dismissed with the label "unsusceptible to sleep."

The ludicrous nature of this example metaphorically illustrates the difficulties in conducting controlled hypnotic research. Experimental results need to be interpreted with caution, and should not bias expectations for future clinical success or failure. Each hypnotic experience is unique and subject to the interaction of numerous extraneous and intrapsychic variables. Standardized inductions prevent the creative therapeutic utilization of these variables and consequently stifle the potential for personal growth and self-discovery.

Erickson succinctly described the inherent difficulties of attempting to create a susceptibility scale that actually measures what it intends to measure: "The unhappy conclusion, briefly stated, is that the whole field of hypnotic research is still so undeveloped that there is very little general understanding either of how to hypnotize a subject satisfactorily for experimental purposes, or of how to elicit the hypnotic phenomena which are to be studied after the subject has been satisfactorily hypnotized" (Erickson & Rossi, 1980, p. 30). He also believed that "the inability of these investigators to replicate each other's findings was due to the poor hypnotic training of their subjects and the researchers' unrealistic expectations about the amount of time, ingenuity, and effort that are actually required to secure valid trance states" (Erickson & Rossi, 1980, p. 299).

It is of particular interest that the codeveloper of the Stanford Scales of Hypnotic Susceptibility, Andre M. Weitzenhoffer, published a report in 1980 which claims: "The Stanford Scales and similar instruments are found to have failed to take into account essential features defining traditional hypnosis and susceptibility and to have created confusion in the scientific inquiry into hypnotism" (p. 130). He discussed the need to modify the use of these scales "if they are to be truly fruitful and valid" (p. 135). He stated that modification should include measurements of enhanced suggestibility, nonvoluntary behavior elicited by suggestion, and spontaneous posthypnotic amnesia. He presented Diamond's (1974) premise that hypnotizability appears to be a learnable skill and hence might be increased with training. Finally, he argued that susceptibility is multidimensional, and that there is a need to distinguish between "clinical" and "laboratory" hypnotizability. Because of these differences, data obtained from one setting "becomes meaningless" when correlated with the other.

SUMMARY

Acceptable scientific research is necessary for the benefits of hypnosis to be further recognized and utilized in the medical and healing fields. However, in order to accurately extrapolate from experimental results, it is necessary to consider the value of each study within its own situational context.

Practical application of experimental conclusions is dependent upon viewing them as flexible guidelines. Research results should be utilized with the clinical intention of expanding on them. This can be done by offering an induction appropriate to the opportunities presented by each individual subject. The reader should be aware that the confines of experimental research should in no way inhibit the creative initiative that so often precedes satisfactory results.

As the reader is now acutely aware, there are some similarities as well as polar extremes existing among some of the major theorists: Spiegel and Erickson, Kroger and Hilgard. While clinical and experimental research has increased and become more sophisticated controversies continue including: what makes for a successful hypnotic induction, what technique is most likely to produce success, whether or not hypnotizeability is important for clinical practice, and whether direct or indirect suggestions are most effective. Furthermore, as stated, the very nature of hypnosis remains unclear.

REFERENCES

Hypnosis Section

Barber, J., & Gitelson, J. (1980). Cancer pain: Psychological management using hypnosis. A *Cancer Journal for Clinicians, 31*, 130–136.

Cousins, N. (1979). Anatomy of an illness as perceived by the patient. New York: W. W. Norton.

Erickson, M. (1952). Deep hypnosis and its induction. In LeCron, L.M. (Ed.), *Experimental hypnosis*. New York: MacMillan.

Erickson, M. (1959). Further clinical techniques of hypnosis: Utilization techniques. *American Journal of Clinical Hypnosis, 2,* 3–21.

Erickson, M., & Rosen, S. (1982). *My voice will go with you.* New York: W. W. Norton & Co.

Erickson, M., Rossi, E., & Rossi, S. (1976). *Hypnotic realities—indirect suggestion.* New York, Irvington, pp. 5–25.

Erickson, M., & Rossi, E. (Eds.) (1980). *Innovative hypnotherapy—The collected papers of Milton H. Erickson on hypnosis Vol. IV.* New York: Irvington.

Erickson, M., & Rossi, E. (1981). *Experiencing hypnosis.* New York: Irvington.

Fromm, E., & Schor, R.(Eds.) (1979). *Hypnosis: Developments in research and new perspectives* (ed. 2). New York: Aldine.

Hilgard, E.R. (1982). Illusion that the eyeroll sign is related to hypnotizability. *Archives of general psychiatry, 39,* 963–966.

Hilgard E.R. (1977). *Divided consciousness: Multiple controls in human thought and action,* New York: Wiley.

Hilgard, E.R. (1979). Divided consciousness in hypnosis: The implications of the hidden observer. In Fromm, E., & Shor, R. (Eds.), *Hypnosis: Developments in research and new perspectives* (ed. 2). New York: Aldine.

Hilgard, E.R., & Hilgard, J.R. (1975). *Hypnosis in the relief of pain,* Lost Altos, CA: William Kauffman.

Holland, B.C. (1967). Discussion: Is symptom removal dangerous? *American Journal of Psychiatry, 123*(10), 1282–1283.

Kroger, W.S. (1977). *Clinical and experimental hypnosis* (ed. 2). Philadelphia: J.B. Lippincott.

Kroger, W.S., & Fezler, W.D. (1976). *Hypnosis and behavior modification: Imagery conditioning.* Philadelphia: J.B. Lippincott.

Melzack, R., & Wall, P.D. (1965). Pain mechanisms: A new theory. *Science,* November 19, 971–979.

Moody, R.A. (1978). *Laugh after laugh—The healing power of humor.* Jacksonville, FL: Headwaters Press.

Moore, R. (1982). Ericksonian theories of hypnosis. *American Journal of Clinical Hypnosis, 24,* 184.

Perry, C., Gelfand R., & Marcovitch, R. (1979). The relevance of hypnotic susceptibility in the clinical context. *Journal of Abnormal Psychology, 88,* 592–603.

Schafer, D., & Hernandez, A. (1978). Hypnosis, pain and the context of therapy. *International Journal of Clinical and Experimental Hypnosis, 26*(3), 143–154.

Spiegel, D., Tryon, W.W., Frischholz, E.J., & Spiegel, H. (1982). Hilgard's illusion (letter). *Archives of General Psychiatry, 39,* 972–974.

Spiegel, H. (1963). The spectrum of hypnotic and non-hypnotic phenomena. *American Journal of Clinical Hypnosis, 4* (1), 1–5.

Spiegel, H. (1967). Is symptom removal dangerous? *American Journal of Psychiatry, 123*(10), 1279–1282.

Spiegel, H. (1972). An eyeroll test for hypnotizability. *American Journal of Clinical Hypnosis, 15,* 25–28.

Spiegel, H. (1974). The grade 5 syndrome: The highly hypnotizable person. *International Journal of Clinical and Experimental Hypnosis*, 22, 303–319.

Spiegel, H. (1974). *Manual for hypnotic induction profile: Eye roll levitation method*, revised. New York: Soni Medica Inc.

Spiegel, H., Spiegel, D. (1978). *Trance and treatment: Clinical uses of hypnosis*. New York: Basic Books.

Vaduro, J., & Butts, P. (1982). Reducing anxiety and pain of childbirth through hypnosis. *American Journal of Nursing*, 82(4), 620–623.

Susceptibility Scales

Barber, J. (1980). Hypnosis and the unhypnotizable. *American Journal of Clinical Hypnosis*. 23, 4–9.

Barber, T.X., & Glass, L.B. (1962). Significant factors in hypnotic behavior. *Journal of Abnormal and Social Psychology*, 64, 222–228.

Barber, T.X., & Wilson S.C. (1979). The Barber suggestibility scale and creative imagination scale: Experimental and clinical applications. *Amiercan Journal of Clinical Hypnosis*, 21, 84–108.

Bentler, P.M., & Hilgard, E.R. (1963). A comparison of group and individual induction of hypnosis with self-scoring and observer-scoring. *International Journal of Clinical Experimental Hypnosis*, 11, 49–54.

Cooper, L., & London, P. (1978–1979). The children's hypnotic susceptibility scale. *American Journal of Clinical Hypnosis*, 21, 170–185.

Erickson, M. (1952). Deep hypnosis and its induction. In LeCron, L.M. (Ed.), *Experimental hypnosis*. New York: Macmillian, 70–114.

Friedlander, J.W., & Sarbin, T.R. (1938). The depth of hypnosis. *Journal of Abnormal and Social Psychology*, 33, 453–475.

Frischholz, E.J., Spiegel, H., Tryon, W.W., & Fischer, S. (1981). The relationship between the hypnotic induction profile and the Stanford hypnotic susceptibility scale, form C: Revisited. *American Journal of Clinical Hypnosis*, 24, 98–105.

Hilgard, E.R. (1965). *Hypnotic susceptibility*. New York: Harcourt, Brace and World.

Hilgard, E.R. (1978–1979). Glossary. *American Journal of Clinical Hypnosis*, 21, 239.

Hilgard, E.R. (1979). The Stanford hypnotic susceptibility scales as related to other measures of hypnotic responsiveness. *American Journal of Clinical Hypnosis*, 21, 68–83.

Hilgard, E.R. (1981). The eyeroll sign and other scores of the hypnotic induction profile (HIP) as related to the Stanford hypnotic susceptibility scales, form C (SHSS:C): A critical discussion of a study by Frischholz and others. *American Journal of Clinical Hypnosis*, 24, 89–97.

Hilgard, E.R. (1981). Further discussion of the HIP and the Stanford form C: A reply to a reply by Frischholz, Spiegel, Tryon and Fisher. *American Journal of Clinical Hypnosis*, 24, 106–108.

Hilgard, E.R., Bowers, P.G., Crawford, H.J., & Kihlstrom, J.F. (1979). A "tailored" SHSS:C, permitting user modification for special purposes. *International Journal of Clinical Hypnosis*, 27, 125–133.

Hilgard, E.R., Weitzenhoffer, A.M., & Gough P. (1958). Individual differences in susceptibility to hypnosis. *Proceedings of the National Academy of Sciences*, 44, 1255–1259.

London, P. (1963). *The children's hypnotic susceptibility scale.* Palo Alto, CA: Consulting Psychologists Press.

Morgan, A.H., & Hilgard, J.R. (1979). The Stanford hypnotic clinical scale: Adult. *American Journal of Clinical Hypnosis, 21,* 134–147.

Morgan, A.H., & Hilgard, J.R. (1979). The Stanford hypnotic clinical scale for children. *American Journal of Clinical Hypnosis, 21,* 148–169.

Shor, R.E., & Orne, E.C. (1962). *Harvard group scale of hypnotic susceptibility.* Palo Alto, CA: Consulting Psychologists Press.

Spiegel, H. (1972). An eyeroll test for hypnotizability. *American Journal of Clinical Hypnosis, 15,* 25–28.

Stern, D.B., Spiegel, H., & Nee, J.C.M. (1978–1979). The hypnotic induction profile: Normative observations, reliability and validity. *American Journal of Clinical Hypnosis, 21,* 109–133.

Weitzenhoffer, A.M. (1983). Hypnotic susceptibility revisited. *American Journal of Clinical Hypnosis, 22,* 130–146.

Weitzenhoffer, A.M., & Hilgard, E.R. (1959). *Stanford hypnotic susceptibility scale, forms A and B,* Palo Alto, CA: Consulting Psychologists Press.

Weitzenhoffer, A.M., & Hilgard, E.R. (1962). *Stanford hypnotic susceptibility scale, form C.* Palo Alto, CA: Consulting Psychologists Press.

Weitzenhoffer, A.M., & Hilgard, E.R. (1963). *Stanford profile scales of hypnotic susceptibility: forms I and II.* Palo Alto, CA: Consulting Psychologists Press.

Weitzenhoffer, A.M., & Hilgard, E.R. (1967). *Revised Stanford profile scales of hypnotic susceptibility, forms I and II.* Palo Alto, CA: Consulting Psychologists Press.

Suggested Readings

Erickson, M., & Rossi, E. (Eds.) (1982). The nature of hypnosis and suggestion: The collected papers of Milton H. Erickson on Hypnosis, Vol. I. New York: Irvington, pp. 15–16.

Erickson, M. (1964). The confusion techniques in hypnosis. *American Journal of Clinical Hypnosis, 6,* 183–207.

Erickson, M. (1958). Naturalistic techniques of hypnosis. *American Journal of Clinical Hypnosis. 1,* 3–8.

Haley, J. (Ed.) (1967). *Advanced techniques of hypnosis and therapy: Selected papers of Milton Erickson, M.D.* New York: Grune & Stratton, p. 2.

Kennedy, M.S. (1983). Hypnosis. In Lego, S. (Ed.), *Lippincott manual of psychiatric/mental health nursing.* Philadelphia: J.B. Lippincott.

Wadden, R.A., & Anderson, C.H. (1982). The clinical use of hypnosis. *Psychological Bulletin, 91*(2), 215–243.

Wain, H.J. (1980). Pain control through use of hypnosis. *American Journal of Clinical Hypnosis, ??,* 41–46.

Wain, H.J. (1979). Hypnosis on a consultation-liaison service. *Psychosomatics, 20*(10), 678–689.

Zahourek, R. (1982). Hypnosis in nursing practice— emphasis on the "problem patient" who has pain (part 1). *Journal of Psychosocial Nursing and Mental Health Service, 20,* 13–17.

3

Therapeutic Suggestion

Dorothy Marie Larkin

The term *suggestion* has been traditionally defined as a stimulus that evokes uncritical acceptance of an idea. This definition tends to create and perpetuate confusion in regard to hypnosis because it implies that the subject is a passive recipient void of capacity to reason. The phrase "uncritical acceptance," misinterpreted, belittles the potential of the subject. The unconscious mind is capable of rejecting any inappropriate or immoral suggestion, but the conscious mind, with all its learned limitations and prejudicial biases, frequently needs to be opened to alternative ideas. This is what effective hypnosis and suggestion can do.

Field (1979) compared the former definition to molding plastic in a machine, and hence referred to it as the mechanistic meaning of suggestion. This approach tends to emphasize the repetitious implantation of ideas via standardized, direct, authoritative suggestions. Passive recipients exposed to such suggestions will typically attribute hypnotic success to the power of the hypnotist. This impression does not afford the subjects warranted personal credit or discovery of their own hypnotic potential.

Another meaning of suggestion was described by Young in 1931, and refers to hinting, indirection, or intimating. Field called this the humanistic aspect of suggestion, because it emphasizes the transactional, mutual aspects of communication. Hypnotized subjects are described as artists who respond to suggested themes and ideas in order to creatively restructure reality (Field, 1979).

Milton Erickson is credited with introducing many of the concepts and freedom of indirect suggestions. He ascribed benefits probably otherwise unattainable to tapping the wisdom of the "doctor within" each individual. "Hypnotic suggestion . . . results in the automatic evocation and utilization of the patient's own unique repertory of response potentials to achieve therapeutic goals that might have been otherwise beyond reach" (Erickson & Rossi, 1981). His suggestions were frequently permissive, open-ended, and replete with options. Most of the Ericksonian literature consists of case studies, since individualized suggestions, inductions, and treatment are difficult to standardize for traditional research.

SUGGESTIBILITY RESEARCH

The scientific literature on suggestibility in hypnosis is extensive and frequently contradictory. Most of the early studies used direct, standardized inductions, and consequently resultant theoretical conclusions are considered potentially valid indicators only when similar direct inductions are utilized.

Pre-1960 data indicate that females are more suggestible than males when a male operator offers the induction (Hilgard et al., 1958; Weitzenhoffer, 1950; Weitzenhoffer & Weitzenhoffer, 1958), but a later study indicates that the sex of the operator makes no significant difference (Hilgard, 1965). Children have been found to be more suggestible than adults, and are believed to be most responsive between the ages of 9 and 12 (London, 1966). Cooper and London (1976) found that children with parents who judged themselves as strict were more suggestible than children with parents who judged themselves as permissive. Responsivity is reportedly established around the age 16, and was found to decline in middle and old age (Berg & Melin, 1975). One report indicates psychoneurotics are more suggestible than emotionally healthy people (Vanderhoof & Clancy, 1962), whereas another concluded that normal subjects are more suggestible than neurotics and psychotics (Hilgard, 1965). A number of studies have found psychotics to be susceptible to suggestion (Abrams, 1964; Friedman & Kleep, 1963; Green, 1969; Ihalainen & Rosberg, 1976; Kramer, 1966; Lavoie et al., 1976).

An important study conducted by Alan Shulik (1979) found that third-person indirect grammatical suggestions significantly increased hypnotic compliance as compared to the traditional second-person direct grammatical suggestions. A standardized susceptibility scale was used to evaluate subject response to second-person grammatical suggestions. A typical example of this type of suggestion is, "You cannot move your arm." The same standardized scale was utilized for comparison, except this scale had the second person "you" changed to third person "she" or "he." Hence, the former sample suggestion would be changed to "She/he cannot move her/his arm." The statistically significant results indicate that indirect wording of inductions facilitates the hypnotic state more than the typical direct inductions. Shulik reasoned that indirect techniques bypass the subject's conscious attitudes and resistances and hence directly influence subject compliance. Erickson similarly utilized this type of indirect technique when he told patients third-person stories that contained relevant solutions to a presenting clinical problem.

TRADITIONAL AND MODERN
THEORIES OF SUGGESTION

Three "Laws of Suggestion" were popularized in 1923 by Emil Coué, and gained further recognition when Kroger republished them in 1977. Although the resilient nature of these principles might imply authenticity, many clinicians consider any law in hypnosis faulty because it does not account for or encourage unique capacities and variations of subject response. Mention is given to these laws because they can enable the modern practitioner to extend basic principles of suggestion beyond preconceived limitations.

The "law of concentrated attention" consists of the premise that "whenever attention is concentrated on an idea over and over again, it spontaneously tends to realize itself" (Kroger, 1977, p. 48). Repetitive radio and television commercials are offered as typical examples of this law. However, it should also be acknowledged that such repetition can backfire, and this author has noted a personal tendency to avoid buying items that are advertised with repellent redundancy. Proponents of Ericksonian hypnosis consider such repetition insulting to the individual's intellect and unconscious mind. These practitioners might instead choose to capture appropriate "concentrated attention" via hints and subtle implications. Many successful advertisers have also reverted to this approach.

The "law of reversed effect" implies that the harder one tries to do something, the less chance one has of success," (Kroger, 1977, p. 48). Kroger reported that continual negative thoughts can lead to their realization because of the belief and expectation that they will happen. This can be true, however, negative thoughts can also lead to creative preventive solutions, and a subject might benefit from viewing a potentially ominous situation in this different light.

The "law of dominant effect" is based on the principle that a strong emotion tends to replace a weaker one. Since the terms "strong" and "weak" are relative concepts, suggestions that effectively divert attention can change their perceptual degree of importance.

Coúe is also credited with the early acknowledgment that generalized, nonspecific suggestions are more successful because they are received with less criticism or resistance. This generalized tendency is exemplified in his famous phrase, "Everyday, in every way, I am getting better and better" (Coué, 1923). His patients, who were encouraged to repeat this phrase several times a day, were then free to choose how they might create desirable change.

Kroger described suggestions as "a process by which sensory impressions are conveyed in a meaningful manner to evoke altered psychophysiologic responses" (Kroger, 1977). Suggestions can provide sensory input via verbal, nonverbal, intraverbal (voice modulation), and extraverbal communication (implication of words). The adept practitioner will utilize each form of communication to offer suggestions in a congruent manner.

Jones (1948) considered effective suggestions to be a composite of three processes: the emotional rapport between subject and facilitator, the acceptance of the suggested idea, and the effect created by the idea once it has been incorporated into the personality.

Weitzenhoffer (1980) described how individuals can respond to suggestions in two different ways. Some subjects will experience their response as voluntary, whereas others perceive the suggested effect involuntarily and without conscious participation. When suggestions bypass higher cortical processes and elicit a nonvoluntary response, it is presumed that unconscious acceptance and participation has been secured.

Kroger (1977) emphasized that suggestibility tendencies (the effect created by suggestion) are significantly determined by the way a subject learned to respond to suggestions in the past. Hence, children, nonassertive adults, and hospitalized patients that have adopted a passive role might initially respond better to suggestions that are offered in a direct, authoritative manner. Therapists can introduce these subjects to the pleasures of independent thinking by gradually offering more suggestions that include choice and require active decision-making.

Other attributes that are frequently considered important in enhancing suggestibility are subject motivation, cooperation, and the capacity to be receptive to new ideas. These variables are subject to change depending on how suggestions are presented to the patient. Therapist ingenuity can ultimately be a more significant dependent factor in securing subject compliance.

WAKING SUGGESTIBILITY AND NURSING IMPLICATIONS

Waking suggestibility consists of an individual's capacity to respond to suggestions without a preliminary trance induction. Although research indicates that suggestibility tends to increase in hypnotic conditions (Weitzenhoffer & Sjoberg, 1961; Hilgard & Tart, 1966), the reported high correlation of hypnotic responsiveness in waking conditions implies that "waking suggestibility may reside within the general domain of hypnosis" (Bowers, K., 1976, p. 89). Furthermore, responding to suggestions can of itself induce a hypnotic trance (Tart, 1970). These results have important implications for the overburdened nurse who might mistakenly believe that hypnotic benefits are realized only when time is available for a formal hypnotic induction. Waking hypnotic suggestions can be interspersed in any nurse–patient conversation, no matter how brief, and tend to compound benefits of other therapeutic interventions.

Recent nursing literature attests to the brevity and ease of utilizing waking suggestions, and emphasizes nurses' capacity to enhance patient compliance (Orndorf & Deutch, 1981; Holderby, 1981). Rogers (1972) described that hospitalized patients are frequently hypersuggestible. Nurses are encouraged to utilize this state of receptivity so patients can be introduced to ideas of a therapeutic and healing nature. She reported that "a patient whose attention is already intensely focused on himself may be in a hypnoidal state during which his suggestibility is so increased that ideas presented to him act like post-hypnotic suggestions" (Rogers, 1972, p. 715).

Whether spontaneous or deliberate, this trance-like state can be recognized when the patient exhibits a sudden fixation of attention and possibly a glassy faraway stare. This is a period when suggestions are more readily accepted because the patient's conscious critical faculties are reduced. The clinician can utilize this receptive state by offering permissive directions, reassurance, and health-promoting education. Assessment should be ongoing. If the subject's attention suddenly shifts, the clinician can concurrently divert her strategy to meet the subject's needs and altered perceptions. When the patient's attention is again secured, suggestions can be offered to further direct awareness toward a therapeutic goal.

SAMPLE SUGGESTION TECHNIQUES

It is initially important to comprehend the difference between direct and indirect suggestions. Most of the traditional inductions available in general hypnosis texts utilize the direct form of suggestion. Minor changes can transform their authoritarian character and create indirect suggestions that will bypass the potential of resistance. The following examples can demonstrate this principle.

DIRECT—Your arm is feeling lighter and lighter and soon it will float off your lap.

INDIRECT—Your arm can feel lighter and lighter and soon it might float off your lap.

INDIRECT—It might be interesting to notice which arm floats off your lap first. I don't know if the lightness will begin at the pinky first and then progress through your hand on up or if it might start with the thumb before the pinky and then move on up. It could even start in a completely different manner or perhaps it might just feel lighter. It really doesn't matter as long as you fully notice the way those changes develop.

The initial indirect change just consisted of rephrasing the suggestion to be more permissive, with the terms "can" and "might."

The second, more developed indirect suggestion conveys a variety of options as to how that lightness might develop. In order for the subject to notice how the implied changes develop, he or she needs to focus inward, which is a desired hypnotic response. Just noticing the changes is also defined as appropriate, so if the arm doesn't go up the subject can still be considered compliant. This type of suggestion is termed fail-safe since any response it evokes will be considered appropriate.

Other methods of phrasing permissive suggestions are, "You *might* be surprised to discover . . . " "*Perhaps* you've already noticed . . . " "You *can* think of *any* pleasant place or time . . . "

CONTINGENT SUGGESTIONS (Erickson & Rossi, 1980. p. 463) are offered by commenting on something that is indisputably true and linking it with something you would like the patient to perceive or experience. "As you take that next breath (the patient will hopefully indisputably take a next breath), *you can begin to notice* further relaxation in that arm."

CONJUNCTIVE SUGGESTIONS (Bandler & Grinder, 1975, p. 20) similarly link two (or three or four) statements but use the term "and." "You're sitting in the chair (indisputably true comment) *and* you can notice something pleasantly different happening to your left hand."

PRESUPPOSITION SUGGESTIONS (Bandler & Grinder, 1975, p. 22) assumes and presupposes a desirable response. "Perhaps you've already noticed a developing sense of numbness in that hand."

CONVERSATIONAL POSTULATES (Bandler & Grinder, 1975, p. 23) typically utilize questions to instruct client behavior. "Can you find a comfortable spot on the wall to focus on?" "Will you sit in this chair to be comfortable?"

DISSOCIATIVE SUGGESTIONS (Erickson & Rossi, 1980, p. 470) can evoke local analgesia by separating perception of a body part or parts. "While *that* leg over *there* continues to heal, you can rest comfortably in the bed." "You can *take your mind* to any pleasant and relaxing scene while we take care of *that* wound." "You can discover a variety of ways to *reorient from the head up.*"

INTERSPERSED SUGGESTIONS (Erickson, 1966) consist of direct suggestions that are interspersed within the framework of a permissive comment or an unrelated statement. "You can *keep on relaxing* George, while I. . . ." "I enjoy sailing too, and it *feels so good, George, so comfortable,* just drifting along wherever the wind might take you." (Erickson's interspersal technique as an induction process is an exquisite testimony of the potential of such suggestions. Curious readers are highly encouraged to obtain and peruse the original reference.)

GENERALIZED REFERENTIAL INDEX (Grinder, Delozier, & Bandler, 1977) describes an actual or hypothetical situation that has direct relevance to the patient and then provides generalized options that the patient can mentally develop. Therapeutic solutions tend to be conveyed in third-person grammatical form and are relayed through stories (Erickson & Rosen, 1982), metaphors (Gordon, D. 1978), and analogies. For example, if the patient is a football player, a story about another football player can effectively secure the patient's attention. Indirect suggestions can then be offered by describing what the first football player did to promote comfort and accelerate the healing process. Erickson frequently prefaced such suggestions with the phrase "I had a patient once who. . . ."

A metaphor that was offered to one of my patients who suffered from severe hypertension consisted of a description of how one learns to drive. Intraverbal voice modulations were utilized to emphasize the italicized suggestions. This example is abbreviated as follows.

> Initially one needs to consciously think about *pressing the brakes* at the *right time* and *when to accelerate properly* so one could arrive *safely* and *comfortably* at the desired destination. But soon the driving *becomes automatic*, with the foot *slowing down* the car or speeding up the car *as appropriate to the situation*, and one can *trust this automatic capacity while enjoying* music on the radio or conversing with a good friend. Now New York taxi drivers are silly in that they speed up so quickly only to stop and wait at the red lights. It seems to much more reasonable to *move along at the proper designated pace* which when *properly timed* can capture all the green lights. . . ."

Subsequent hourly vital signs indicated normal blood pressure for the remainder of the shift, and the subject gleefully reported that she learned how to make it automatic. Since her medications were ordered according to specific blood pressure parameters, it wasn't necessary to secure a prescription change.

POSTHYPNOTIC SUGGESTIONS are suggestions offered during hypnosis that are intended to be carried out in the subsequent waking state. The suggested response is usually elicited by an associated cue, and tends to spontaneously reinstate a brief hypnotic trance (Udoff, 1981, pp. 143–144): "When the doctor comes to check that wound, you can be surprised at how quickly you relax and be comfortable. . . ."

SUGGESTIONS FOR REORIENTATION FROM TRANCE should reverse any suggested effect that is not appropriate for maintaining in the waking state. "As you reorient, that numbness can change to comfort, and it can stay that way as long as proper healing continues." (This suggestion safely ensures comfort unless healing is not progressing properly, in which case the subject will need to attend to the resultant lack of comfort and seek proper medical attention.)

Since this hypnotic state is so pleasant, subjects frequently appreciate a few minutes of "world time" to reorient. "Take two or three minutes of world time to comfortably finish for now what you've already begun, knowing full well that you can return to this state at any proper time, perhaps just by taking three deep breaths. After that world time you can reorient alert, refreshed and possibly delighted. . . ."

NONTHERAPEUTIC SUGGESTIONS AND
COUNTERING MEASURES

The beginning practitioner will also discover a variety of opportunities to counter nontherapeutic suggestions. Frequently, these hurtful suggestions are given to patients by well-meaning professionals who are unaware of the potential maladaptive impact of their communications. A professional's benevolent intent of truthfully conveying to patients probable perceptions of medical procedures is legally warranted and ethically appropriate, but too often the negative potential response is emphasized at the expense of potentially positive or neutral responses. For example, in my practice with burn patients, it was necessary to dress the wounds with an antibiotic that was frequently perceived as uncomfortably hot. Other nurses would often warn patients with statements like, "Get ready, because this dressing is going to burn." Naturally, the patients would apprehensively pay attention to the predicted burning sensation, and subsequently complained or grimaced when the heat was felt. When I dressed patients with this topical antiobiotic, I truthfully told them that, "This dressing is going to feel wet" (a simultaneous perceptual experience). The occasional patient who did report discomfort from excessive warmth would have that experience accepted and acknowledged* and then I would suggestively redirect attention to another different truthful perceptual experience, perhaps toward the concept of time, with "Yes, but most patients say the heat lasts only a short time, and I wonder *how soon yours will quit* (interspersed suggestion for brevity of discomfort)."

Another burn patient was scheduled for his first post-operative burn cleansing tank immersion procedure. His attending physician loudly announced within the patient's hearing range, "Get the thrombin ready, *he was just debrided and he's going to lose a lot of blood.*" To counter this nontherapeutic conjunctive suggestion, I calmly but emphatically stated at his ear level, "Although, I wonder how interesting it might be to *notice how little you need to bleed,* perhaps *just the amount needed to clean the burns properly, so they can heal even quicker.* After all, you have been *stopping the bleeding* all your life, and even if you don't fully understand how to do it, *you do know how to do it,* and maybe you could just *watch to see how it's done properly this time. . . .*" (element of confusion technique* with indirect suggestion to let the unconscious mind direct the process). These suggestions were subtly reemphasized throughout the procedure and were interspersed with suggestions for relaxation, deep breathing, and enhanced comfort. The patient was compliant, relaxed, and required very little thrombin.

Another example of countering nontherapeutic suggestions was when a 9

---

*See Utilization Techniques, p. 31, Larkin's section on Ericksonian hypnosis, Chapter 2.
*See Confusion Technique, p. 31–32, Larkin's section on Ericksonian approaches in hypnosis in Chapter 2.

year-old dying leukemic boy with a variety of IV lines and tubes, Swan and arterial line monitors, respirator and chest tubes needed to be log-rolled and weighed. An attending nurse informed the boy that she was sorry, but this was going to hurt him. The patient responded with a grimace and a moan. The author then commented that "Sometimes it *can be more comfortable* if one *moves slowly, carefully, and gently,* and maybe *takes a few slow deep breaths, which can really help.*" His furrowed brow relaxed, and he took a deep breath and began to assist us by slowly moving one arm and leg. The other nurse responded with, "Oh, no, there's no way you can be comfortable log-rolling with a chest tube. Chest tubes always make you hurt." The boy's frown and grimace returned. The author countered with, "I'm not so sure about that, but it might be really interesting to *find out how comfortable it could be . . . , with deep breaths, and slow careful movements, right now . . . , so maybe the hurt won't even need to bother him.*" The patient's forehead again relaxed and he proceeded to assist us further. The other nurse was verbally persistent in maintaining her position that comfort could not exist, and the conversation continued to offer the patient opposing suggestions (to which the patient correspondingly alternated relaxed and furrowed brow) until the author chose to monopolize the conversation. The procedure was completed with willing patient participation and minimal nonverbal indications of discomfort.

The scope of this chapter only permits a preliminary introduction to the process of formulating effective suggestions. References are provided and workshops are available for further elaboration and concept clarification. However, the more comprehensive form of education will occur as the clinician observes patients' verbal and nonverbal responses to therapeutic suggestions. This is when the value of this adjunctive tool truly becomes apparent.

REFERENCES

Abrams, S. (1964). The use of hypnotic techniques with psychotics, a critical review. *American Journal of Psychotherapy, 18,* 79.

Bandler, R., & Grinder, J. (1975). *Patterns of the hypnotic techniques of Milton H. Erickson, M.D. (vol. 1).* Cupertino, CA: Meta Publications.

Berg, S., & Melin, E. (1975). Hypnotic susceptibility in old age: Some data from residential homes for old people. *International Journal of Clinical and Experimental Hypnosis, 23,* 184.

Bowers, K. (1976). *Hypnosis for the seriously curious.* Belmont, CA: Wadsworth Publishing.

Cooper, L.M., & London, P. (1976). Children's hypnotic susceptability personality and EEG patterns. *International Journal of Clinical and Experimental Hypnosis, 24*(2), 140–148.

Coué, E. (1923). *Hos to practice suggestion and autosuggestion.* New York: American Library Service.

Diamond, M.J. (1974). Issues and methods for modifying responsivity to hypnosis, *Annals of the New York Academy of Sciences*, 296, 119–128.

Erickson, M. (1966). The interspersal hypnotic technique for symptom correction and pain control. *American Journal of Clinical and Experimental Hypnosis*, 3, 198–209.

Erickson, M., & Rosen, S. (1982). *My voice will go with you*. New York: W.W. Norton & Co.

Erickson, M., & Rossi, E. (Ed.) (1980). *The collected papers of Milton H. Erickson, volume 1—The nature of hypnosis and suggestion*. New York: Irvington Publications.

Erickson, M., & Rossi, E. (1981). *Experiencing hypnosis—Therapeutic approaches to altered states*. New York: Irvington Publications.

Field, P.B. (1979). Humanistic aspects of hypnotic communication. In Fromm, E., & Shor, R. (Eds.). *Hypnosis: Developments in research and new perspectives, (ed. 2)*., New York: Aldine Publishing, pp. 609–610.

Friedman, J., & Kleep, W. (1963). Hypnotizability of newly admitted psychotic patients. *Psychosomatics*, 4, 95.

Green, J.T. (1969). Hypnotizability of hospitalized psychotics. *International Journal of Clinical and Experimental Hypnosis*, 17, 103.

Gordon, D. (1978). Therapeutic metaphors. Cupertino, CA: Meta Publishing.

Grinder, J., Delozier, J., & Bandler, R. (1977). *Patterns of the hypnotic techniques of Milton H. Erickson, M.D., vol. 2*. Cupertino, CA: Meta Publications.

Hilgard, E.R., Weitzenhoffer, A.M., & Gough, P., et al. (1958). Individual differences in susceptibility to hypnosis. *Proceedings of the National Academy of Sciences*, 44, 1255–1259.

Hilgard, E.R. (1965). *Hypnotic susceptibility*. New York: Harcourt, Brace & World.

Hilgard, E.R., & Tart, C.J. (1966). Responsiveness to suggestions following waking and imagination instructions and following induction of hypnosis. *Journal of Abnormal Psychology*, 71, 196–208.

Holderby, R. (1981). Conscious suggestions: Using talk to manage pain. *Nursing*, 11, 44–46.

Ihalainen, O., & Rosberg, G. (1976). Relaxing and encouraging suggestions given to hospitalized chronic schizophrenics. *International Journal of Clinical and Experimental Hypnosis*, 24, 228.

Jones, E. (1978). The nature of auto-suggestion: In *Papers on psycho-analysis* (ed. 5). Baltimore: Williams & Wilkins.

Kramer, E. (1966). Group induction of hypnosis with institutionalized patients. *International Journal of Clinical and Experimental Hypnosis*, 14, 243.

Kroger, W.S. (1977). *Clinical and experimental hypnosis*, (2nd Ed.). Philadelphia: J.B. Lippincott.

Lavoie, G., Sabourin, M., Ally, G., & Langlois, J. (1976). Hypnotizability as a function of adoptive regression among chronic psychotic patients. *International Journal of Clinical and Experimental Hypnosis*, 3, 238.

London, P. (1966). Child hypnosis and personality. *American Journal of Clinical Hypnosis*, 8, 161.

Orndorf, R., & Deutch, J. (1981). The power of positive suggestion—persuading patients to cooperate. *Nursing*, 11, 73.

Rogers, B. (1972). Therapeutic conversation and posthypnotic suggestion. *American Journal of Nursing*, 72, 714–717.

Shulik, A. M. (1979). Right versus left hemispheric communication styles in hypnotic inductions and the facilitation of hypnotic trance. *Dissertation Abstracts International, 40,* p. 2445-B.

Spiegel, H., & Bridger, A. A. (1970). Manual for hypnotic induction profile: Eye roll-levitation method. New York: Basic Books, 1.

Tart, C.J. (1970). Self-report scales of hypnotic depth. *International Journal of Clinical and Experimental Hypnosis, 18,* 105–125.

Udolf, R. (1981). *Handbook of hypnosis for professionals.* New York: Van Nostrand Reinhold.

Vanderhoof, E., & Clancy, J. (1962). Effect of emotion on blood flow. *Journal of Applied Physiology, 17,* 67.

Weitzenhoffer, A. (1950). A note on the persistence of hypnotic suggestion. *Journal of Abnormal and Social Psychology, 45,* 160.

Weitzenhoffer, A. (1980). Hypnotic susceptibility revisited. *American Journal of Clinical Hypnosis, 22,* 130–146.

Weitzenhoffer, A., & Sjoberg, B. (1961). Suggestibility with and without induction of hypnosis. *Journal of Nervous and Mental Disease, 132,* 205–220.

Weitzenhoffer, A.M., & Weitzenhoffer, G.B. (1958). Personality and hypnotic susceptibility. *American Journal of Clinical Hypnosis, 1,* 79.

Young, P.C. (1931). Suggestion as Indirection. *Journal of Abnormal and Social Psychology, 26,* 69–90.

4

Legal, Religious, and
Professional Issues*

Ronald L. McBride

This chapter will discuss areas of concern that occur frequently in the employment of hypnosis. No attempt will be made to completely describe all of the details of the major positions, as such an undertaking would result in a chapter many times the size of this entire book. Hence, the material in this chapter will be presented summarily, with the major emphasis on practicalities.

LEGAL ISSUES

Litigation involving hypnosis is rare, and as a result there is very little case law on the subject. Of those cases coming to court, the most common claims have been that hypnosis was used to induce a client to commit a crime or to victimize the client.

Knowing what hypnosis is and is not, it is difficult to believe that it could be used to induce a client to commit a crime if he or she is not ordinarily so inclined. Most authorities believe the hypnotherapist has no power to compel a client to commit any act that would be repugnant or that would go against the client's moral, ethical, or religious beliefs. Suggestions are only effective if they are acceptable to the client.* A client in hypnosis is not unconscious, and is

---

*Editors notes: This chapter utilizes nursing examples. Legal vagaries and restricted membership in hypnosis associations apply to other disciples as well and are currently being discussed in the associations.

*During times of extreme duress (i.e., war) people are more susceptible to suggestions that may not fit their normal moral code, according to Kroger (1977). It is *conceivable* for an unscrupulous hypnotist to produce amnesia, establish a valid motive, and propel an individual into an antisocial act. This, however, is not part of a therapeutic relationship.

aware of his or her surroundings and of what is being said to him or her. It would be unlikely the client could be deceived or convinced to commit a criminal or antisocial act. Even in the deepest stage of hypnosis—the somnambulistic state—there is no loss of consciousness or reflexes, although there is some alteration of awareness and posthypnotic amnesia.

To elicit antisocial, immoral, or criminal behavior through hypnotic suggestion requires (1) altering the client's perception of that behavior and (2) misleading the client into believing that such behavior would be justified and without consequence. To produce such behavior in an unsuspecting client would be a paramount misuse of hypnosis. The liability of an unethical hypnotherapist who suggests such behavior is unquestionable and would be guilty of criminal solicitation, accessory before the fact, and/or conspiracy.

Using hypnosis to victimize a client is another area of concern. This may involve sexual molestation/seduction or the attempt to influence the client for financial or other advantageous favors. The former is the most common accusation. As with induced criminal behavior, it is difficult to believe that this is possible. However, there have been reported cases of a hypnotherapist having sexual relations with a hypnotized client. If a court were convinced that hypnotic suggestion had caused the patient to submit to sexual relations, this would be regarded as the equivalent of force and the hypnotherapist would be guilty of rape. Sexual relations between any therapist and patient is both malpractice and unprofessional conduct.

The possibility of an ethical hypnotherapist being falsely accused of such behavior should also be considered. Dr. Udolf (1981) points out that people who violate standards of professional conduct do so time after time. So, it would be difficult to believe that a previously ethical and professional hypnotherapist would suddenly depart from customary professional conduct. Fortunately this type of accusation is quite rare. However, there have been reports of clients who have fantasized a sexual assault by the hypnotherapist. The hypnotherapist should take some elementary measures to minimize the possibility of an occurrence. During the intial interview and evaluation, the therapist should carefully note any apparent severe maladjustment or erotic fantasies. If the client is of the opposite sex and the hypnotherapist feels there is a potential problem, a third party should be present or in the next room. Making a tape recording of the session will inhibit a patient from making false charges of misconduct. Voice tone and inflection should be carefully self-monitored by the hypnotherapist in order to avoid sounding unctious or seductive. Remember that an impeccable professional reputation is the best protection against claims of unethical conduct.

LEGISLATIVE ISSUES

Little federal and state legislation exists relating to the teaching of hypnosis or to the regulation of who may use it in therapeutic situations. Most attempted legislation has been aimed at the elimination of stage hypnosis for entertainment. Other attempts have been proposed by professional groups seeking to restrict the use of hypnosis to only that particular profession. Since hypnosis is considered a safe procedure when used by a trained clinician, it should not be legislated as the exclusive property of any particular group. One reason legislators have found it difficult to draft legislation that is effective and fair is that hypnosis involves nothing more than one person talking to another. Furthermore, hypnosis is a natural phenomenon that can occur spontaneously without formal induction. Therefore, it is nearly impossible and rather impractical to attempt to control it legislatively.

Within the United States, there is no state that prohibits the practice of hypnosis by law or statute. The majority have no legislation whatsoever relating to hypnosis. Of those that do, the laws are somewhat outdated and relate mostly to prohibiting hypnosis for entertainment or are loose attempts at regulating who may practice hypnosis and hypnotherapy. For example, Kansas Statute Section 21-4007 makes "Hypnotic Exhibition" a class C misdemeanor. "No one can give for entertainment any instruction, demonstration or performance in which hypnosis is used or is attempted." A Florida law (Chapter 456) reads, "It shall be unlawful for any person to engage in the practice of hypnosis for therapeutic purposes unless such person is a practitioner of one of the healing arts, as herein defined, or acts under supervision, direction, prescriptions and responsibility of such a person."

Aside from state laws and statutes, there may be state Medical Practice Acts, Psychology Practice Acts, and/or Nursing Practice Acts that would have jurisdiction over nurses using hypnosis. The following statement comes from the New Hampshire Attorney General: "It has been determined by the Board of Registration in Medicine that hypnosis and hypnotherapy are part of the practice of medicine and can be performed only by someone who is licensed to practice medicine in this state." Checking various states' Nurse Practice Acts, none were found that prohibit nurses from using hypnosis, nor is there any law prohibiting a nurse from encouraging increased relaxation or using suggestions purposefully to a therapeutic end. A few, such as the Colorado Nurse Practice Act specifically allows nurses to utilize hypnosis.

RELIGIOUS ISSUES

Many religions of the world utilize meditation, chanting, and prayers to "open up the mind" or produce serenity and tranquility within the body. This narrowing and focusing of attention during such practices produces a state of relaxation.

The only major religious groups in the United States that discourage their members from using hypnosis are Seventh Day Adventists, Christian Scientists, and Jehovah Witnesses. They admit that hypnosis has medical value when performed by a qualified practitioner, but they prefer their members to utilize techniques and methods taught by the particular church. Looking closely at their methods of "healing through the mind," one can see they are actually utilizing hypnosis and hypnotic techniques. They simply do not wish to refer to it as such. No other major religions have restrictions for using hypnosis. In fact, several have made statements of an official nature in support of the value of hypnosis when used properly by a trained practitioner.

Many other practices such as yoga, transcendental meditation, Silva mind control, and biofeedback differ from hypnosis merely in name. Individuals who practice any of the above would make excellent hypnotic subjects since they are already conditioned to the relaxed state.

ETHICAL AND PROFESSIONAL ISSUES

The first prerequisite to becoming an ethical and professional hypnotherapist is to receive adequate education and training in hypnosis. Care should be exercised in selecting a program or school, because there are probably as many who are interested only in getting money as there are those who are interested in giving students a good, basic, comprehensive education in hypnotherapy. Reputable schools are approved by the state or other accrediting organization. After completing formal education it is important to continue to learn everything there is to know relating to the chosen area of practice. Diplomas and certificates should be openly displayed so that clients may examine them. This helps gain client confidence and demonstrates the therapist's qualifications.

More and more workshops and courses are being conducted across the country by and for nurses. Many of the authors of chapters in the book are engaged in that endeavor; the reader is encouraged to seek out these workshops from nurses as well as other professionals to augment their reading and expand their practice.

A professional appearance and approach to patients are important. The first impression will be a lasting one, and good rapport is essential to successful hypnotherapy.

A good hypnotherapist is aware of contraindications in the use of hypnosis. Any client who shows evidence of severe depression, suicidal tendencies, prepsychosis, or psychosis should be referred to a psychotherapist. The clinician should also be aware of personal limitations. For example, if working with clients who have sexual problems makes the therapist uncomfortable or if knowledge of treating such problems is limited, such cases should not be accepted.

The use of advertising should be limited and very professional. Usually a simple listing in the yellow pages is adequate. Never use tasteless ads that make false or unrealistic claims.

Membership in at least one professional hypnosis organization is highly recommended, as is subscribing to professional publications. The following list of organizations is provided simply as a starting point and does not necessarily indicate any endorsement. Some of the organizations listed have restricted memberships but have been included because they have excellent publications. One would need to contact the organizations directly for membership and publication information.

1. Association to Advance Ethical Hypnosis, Power Publishers, Inc., 60 Voss Ave., South Orange, NJ 07079.
2. The American Institute of Hypnosis, 7188 Sunset Blvd., Los Angeles, CA 90046.
3. International Society for Professional Hypnosis, 218 Monroe Street, Boonton, NJ 07005.
4. International Society for Clinical and Experimental Hypnosis, 111 North 49th Street, Philadelphia, PA 19139.
5. Society for Clinical and Experimental Hypnosis, 129 A Kings Park Drive, Liverpool, NY 13088.
6. American Society of Clinical Hypnosis, 2400 East Devon Avenue, Suite 218, Des Plains, IL 60018.
7. American Guild of Hypnotherapists, Medical Division, 1021 North Carrollton Avenue, New Orleans, LA 70119.

The American Guild of Hypnotherapists is a little different from the other organizations listed in that it is not an organization per se but rather a registry and referral service. Membership in the Medical Division is limited to those in the health care professions and is based on hypnosis education and qualification. Membership allows the individual to legally use the initials "R.H." (Registered Hypnotherapist) following one's name. The Guild maintains an up-to-date listing of members so that referrals can be made throughout the United States. They also publish a quarterly journal.

Many professional issues confront the nurse. These are alluded to in the first chapter (overview) and need expansion here. On occasion, because of mythology associated with hypnosis a physician, nurse college, or supervisor will be reluctant to allow the nurse to utilize hypnosis. The nurse, armed with knowledge in this book, workshop or specialized training, and supervision is best able to counter the misconceptions and allay fears that hypnosis is dangerous out of the realm of nursing or in the realm of the occult or magical.

CONCLUSION

When nurses use hypnosis solely within their nursing practice it is simply another nursing tool. As nurses are licensed health care professionals, there is usually no conflict with regulatory agencies. However, the nurse who opens a private hypnotherapy practice becomes responsible for consulting with the State Board of Nursing and observing any and all regulatory laws and statutes governing hypnosis in that jurisdiction.

Maintaining the highest professional and ethical standards is the most valuable contribution nurses can make to the progress and acceptance of hypnosis.

SUGGESTED READINGS

Barber, T.X. (1961). Antisocial and criminal acts induced by "hypnosis": A review of experimental and clinical findings. *Archives of General Psychiatry*, 5:301–312.

Bryan, W.J., Jr. (1962). *Legal aspects of hypnosis*. Springfield, IL: Charles C. Thomas.

Coe, W.C., Kobayashi, K., & Howard, M.L. (1972). An approach toward isolating factors that influence antisocial conduct in hypnosis. *International Journal of Clinical and Experimental Hypnosis, 20*, 118–131.

Erickson, M.H. (1939). An experimental investigation of the possible antisocial use of hypnosis. *Psychiatry, 2*, 391–414.

Hammerschlag, H.E. (1957). *Hypnotism and crime*. Hollywood: Wilshire Book Co.

Kline, M.V. (1972). The production of antisocial behavior through hypnosis: New clinical data. *International Journal of Clinical and Experimental Hypnosis, 20*(2), 80–94.

Kroger, W.S. (1977). Clinical and experimental hypnosis in medicine, dentistry and psychology. 2nd ed. Philadelphia: J.B. Lippincott.

McCoy, L.R. (1973). *Professional hypnology course manual*. New Orleans: Academy of Clinical Hypnosis.

O'Brien, R.M., & Rabuck, S.J. (1976). Experimentally proposed self-repugnant behavior as a function of hypnosis and waking suggestion: A pilot study. *American Journal of Clinical Hypnosis, 18*(4), 272–276.

Orne, M.T. (1965). Can a hypnotized subject be compelled to carry out otherwise unacceptable behavior? *International Journal of Clinical and Experimental Hypnosis, 13*(4), 226–237.

Udolf, R. (1981). *Handbook of hypnosis for professionals*. New York: Van Nostrand Reinhold.

—————————————— 5 ——————————————

Stress and Coping: Working with the Well Population *

Carolyn Chambers Clark

Hypnotic techniques (imagery, relaxation and suggestion) can be used by nurses when working with a relatively well population. The word "relatively" seems most appropriate because even when no disease processes are evident, factors such as stress, lack of fitness, the environment, lack of positive relationships, lack of life purpose, or insufficient knowledge regarding self-care practices interact to set the stage for a less than totally well individual (Clark, 1981a). When working with such an individual, it is up to the nurse to assess internal indicators that warn of excessive stress or lack of wellness, and to teach the client to do the same. The chief purpose of assessment and intervention with the well population is to locate warning signals via imagery and use individualized prescriptions to help the client return to a higher level of wellness. Imagery and inner dialogue techniques are especially well suited to this purpose.

CLIENT PREPARATION

The first step is to assist the client to attain total body relaxation or a good approximation thereof. There are a number of methods of attaining this goal (see Chapter 3). Some clients relax more readily with one approach than another; it is up to the nurse to observe and collaborate with each client to find the relaxation technique (or combination of techniques) most useful for attain-

Research supported in part by a grant from the Robert Wood Johnson Foundation Grant to the Lienhard School of Nursing Research and Clinical Practice Unit for Faculty Practice and Research, and by a Pace University Scholarship Research Grant.

*Editors note: The reader who is not a nurse is encouraged to substitute the word clinician for nurse as it appears throughout this chapter.

61

ing a relaxed state. Initially, the nurse may read a prepared relaxation script, play a relaxation audiotape or repeat a useful relaxation monologue. A relatively simple and quick way to attain relaxation by altering the client's consciousness state is to make comments to put the client in touch with what is being experienced through various sensory modes but is out of total awareness (Grinder & Bandler, 1981). For example, if a client is sitting with her hands on her thighs and her feet on the floor, the nurse might say, "You can become aware of the feeling of your hands on your thighs and the sensation of your feet on the floor." A second method involves assisting the client to take an inner journey to a peaceful, quiet, relaxing place. In this case, the nurse might say, "Close your eyes and take yourself in your mind's eye to a peaceful, quiet, relaxing place. Immerse yourself in that place, smelling the smells, hearing the sounds, seeing what there is to see, feeling all the sensations available to you there."

Although the nurse provides the content for the relaxation at first, by the end of the first session the nurse teaches the client an appropriate relaxation method and encourages out-of-session practice to attain a state of relaxation. Some nurses make audiotapes for clients to use between sessions, others give clients relaxation scripts or encourage them to develop their own regimen for daily practice. Whichever method is used, it is suggested to the client that relaxation is a learned skill that requires regular, systematic practice.

USE OF SUGGESTION FOR STRESS REDUCTION

There are two ways to use suggestion for stress reduction. The first includes the following steps: (1) obtain data regarding the client problem, (2) agree on an individualized stress reduction suggestion, (3) assist the client to a relaxed state, (4) repeat and/or ask the client to repeat the stress reduction suggestion.

The second approach includes the same steps, but reorders them, placing the client in a relaxed state at the beginning of the session. In this case, the nurse and client can agree on finger signals prior to beginning the relaxation procedures. For example, the nurse can ask the client to "raise the index finger of your right (or left) hand when you feel completely relaxed" and "raise the little finger of your right (or left) hand when you feel yourself becoming less relaxed."

This approach allows the nurse to stop assessment questions that induce stress and proceed directly to a relaxation procedure until stress is reduced and assessment can continue. This procedure alone is often helpful in reducing the client's anxiety level sufficiently to preclude the use of further intervention.

The order of intervention chosen is based on a number of factors, including (1) level of client resistance to use of suggestion; (2) level of client comfort with each order of intervention; (3) level of nurse resistance to use of suggestion; and (4) level of nurse comfort with each order of intervention.

Once the stressful situation has been identified, it may be necessary for the nurse and client to spend some time deciding which portion of the situation to focus on and how the suggestions can be worded most effectively for that client. For example, in a situation in which a student becomes highly anxious while taking an examination, the suggestion could be focused on relaxing the student, reducing the threat of the examination questions or environment, or both. Some suggestions that may be appropriate include, "I will pass this exam" (self-focused); "These questions are questions I know the answer to" (environment-focused); "I can become more relaxed and focus on the exam questions" (both).

DESIGNING STRESS REDUCTION SUGGESTIONS

To get the flavor of how stress reduction suggestions can be formulated, examine the stressful client situations below and think of a suggestion to use for each client.

1. Fear of being alone in the house at night
2. Feeling anxious about work or school deadlines but being unable to concentrate
3. Being unable to get to sleep
4. Feelings of being inferior to classmates or work peers
5. Worry about being rejected for a job, a grade, or a date

Now, examine some possible suggestions for the above situations:

1. It's getting easier and easier to stay home alone at night.
2. I'm getting more and more relaxed about getting my work done and/or it's getting easier and easier to concentrate on the task at hand.
3. I'm gradually becoming more drowsy and in a few minutes I'll be able to fall asleep.
4. Each time I'm with _____ it's getting easier and easier to feel relaxed and good about myself.
5. By letting my breath flow through me I can feel confidence flowing throughout my whole body.

USING STRESS COPING THOUGHTS

Another stress reduction approach that can also be used by clients for self-care purposes is teaching stress coping thoughts (Davis, McKay, & Eschelman, 1980). Their approach is based on cognitive psychology theory, which holds that thoughts rule feelings: the way the future or present is imagined intensifies or decreases the feelings experienced.

For example, if a bus is missed, the person can negatively interpret the situation thinking, "Oh, dear, now I'm late, I'll never get all my work done," or positively interpret by thinking, "Well, now I have a few minutes to relax and enjoy the scenery and the people." The first interpretation will probably lead to knots in the stomach, increased heart rate, and so on. The second interpretation will probably lead to decreased heart and respiratory rate and feelings of calmness, if not enjoyment.

When working to reverse negative thoughts, there are suggestions the client can learn to use at each phase of the stressful situation. Anticipating the stressful event, the client could say: "I'm going to be all right," "I won't let this upset me," or "I've handled this situation before and gotten through it all right." At the beginning of a stressful situation, suggestions such as the following can be used: "I'll take this step by step," "I'm doing my best and I'll be okay," and "I'm getting tense and so I'll focus on taking some deep, relaxing breaths." When the situation ends, the client can say, "I got through it and I did well," "I'm able to handle this situation," or "I'm going to tell one other person how well I did."

The most effective coping thoughts are probably those developed by the client, and these suggestions can provide guidelines for formulation for future activities. Once coping thoughts have been formulated, clients can write them on 3 x 5 cards, carry them with them, and read them when confronted with a stressful situation.

HELPING CLIENTS REFUTE IRRATIONAL IDEAS

Irrational thinking creates stress because the person feels things are being done *to* him or her, and a sense of mastery over one's destiny is lost. Rational thinking assists people to perceive that (1) events happen in the world; (2) these events can be viewed as positive, negative or neutral experiences; and (3) positive, neutral, or negative feelings are experienced as a result of how a situation is viewed.

Davis, McKay and Eschelman (1980) suggested the following format for refuting irrational ideas:

1. Write down the event that led to a loss of sense of mastery (e.g., "I failed an exam").
2. Write down any rational ideas about the event that indicate understanding another point of view or the blamelessness of the situation (e.g., "I didn't study").
3. Write down any irrational ideas that indicate that something is being done to you or that loss of control, confidence, or self-esteem has occurred (e.g., "The teacher is out to get me").
4. Write down any feelings that resulted from the irrational ideas (e.g., "I feel angry and depressed").

5. Challenge any irrational ideas (e.g., "I'm not the only one who failed so he can't be out to get just me; I've talked myself into getting depressed; the worst thing that can happen is I won't get an A in the course, but it doesn't mean I'm a bad person").

6. Make concrete plans for dealing rationally with the situation (e.g., "I'll have to study harder to get a better grade; I'll treat myself to a good dinner and then talk with a friend awhile until I feel better. I'm beginning to feel better already.").

The principles of effective suggestion are practiced whether the nurse works with the well or ill population. These principles include the following:

1. Make statements positive ("I'm becoming more relaxed" rather than "I am not tense").

2. Formulate statements in a becoming mode ("I'm becoming more relaxed" rather than "I am relaxed").

3. Keep statements brief and focused specifically on goals.

4. Use repetition, saying the statement five or more times at least three times a day (Curtis & Detert, 1981).

TEACHING CLIENTS TO USE A
STRESS REDUCTION HIERARCHY

Everyone encounters stressful situations. Relaxation can be combined with imagery to reduce the threat posed by stress through the use of a stress reduction hierarchy. As with other approaches, effective relaxation skills form the basis for use of stress reduction hierarchies (Davis, McKay & Eschelman, 1980). Once the client is able to relax at will, the nurse and client formulate a stress hierarchy for the dreaded situation. For example, suppose the dreaded event is speaking up in an interdisciplinary conference. The end goal is speaking up in the conference. Yet, there are a series of preceding steps the client must move through in order to be relaxed in the situation. The first step is to attain total body relaxation (Table 5-1). Using this hierarchy as an example, the nurse can work with the client in the following ways:

1. Agree on finger signals for increased and decreased relaxation.

2. Assist the client to a relaxed state.

3. Move from one step to the next only when the client signals a deep state of body relaxation.

4. Whenever decreased relaxation is signalled, assist the client to attain a deeply relaxed state, watching the client's finger signals to indicate when to move to the next step.

5. Work back and forth between assisting the client to relax and moving closer to the end goal until the client feels relaxed imagining the goal.

Table 5-1. A Hierarchy of Practice Experiences to Attain the End Goal: Speaking Up in an Interdiscipinary Conference

---

End Goal: Picturing yourself speaking up in an interdisciplinary conference while feeling relaxed.

Step 15: As in Step 3.

Step 14: Picturing yourself waiting for your chance to speak up in the conference.

Step 13: As in Step 3.

Step 12: Picturing yourself entering the room and being seated.

Step 11: As in Step 3.

Step 10: Picturing yourself approaching the door of the conference room.

Step 9: As in Step 3.

Step 8: Picturing yourself on the way to the interdisciplinary conference.

Step 7: As in Step 3.

Step 6: Picturing yourself dressing and thinking about speaking up in the conference.

Step 5: As in Step 3.

Step 4: Picturing yourself getting out of bed and thinking about speaking up in the interdisciplinary conference.

Step 3: Check for decreased relaxation; if anxiety has risen, stop that image and return to total body relaxation method until relaxation is attained, then move back one image and proceed.

Step 2: Picturing yourself waking up and remembering today is the day to speak up in the interdisciplinary conference.

Step 1: Attain total body relaxation.

---

6. Suggest to the client that now body, thoughts, and feelings are integrated in a relaxed, whole way, making it easier and easier to relax in the actual situation when it occurs.

A different client may develop a different hierarchy; fewer steps may be involved, or more may be added, depending on the level of stress attached to the event. Regardless of the number of steps involved, the progression remains the same. In this approach, as in the others mentioned, check back and forth with the client to ensure the appropriate number of steps are used and words relevant to the client's experience are chosen.

USING GUIDED IMAGERY WITH CLIENTS

There are three basic ways to use imagery with clients (Samuels and Samuels, 1975):

1. Receptive—to help become more aware of feelings, dissatisfactions, tensions, and images that are affecting body functioning.

2. Healing—to help erase bacteria or viruses, build new cells to replace damaged ones, make rough areas smooth, hot areas cool, sore areas comfortable, tense areas relaxed, drain swollen areas, release pressure from tight areas, bring blood to areas that need nutriment or cleansing, make moist areas dry or dry areas moist, bring energy to fatigued areas, and enhance general wellness.
3. Problem solving—to consult with one's intuitive source of wisdom in a structured way.

Each of these will be discussed in turn.

Receptive Guided Imagery

Research is currently being conducted by the author to investigate whether nursing student clients have intuitive knowledge about their bodies that is not currently being assessed by traditional nursing assessment procedures. Diagnostic Guided Imagery is the tool being used to measure this intuitive knowledge.

Since the conscious mind is bypassed when using imagery, this approach can move a client easily to uncovering strong feelings. Because of this, an occasional client may seem confused by the strong feelings experienced. It is wise to suggest to clients that they need only become aware of feelings they feel comfortable handling at that time. Such a comment reduces resistance to becoming aware of feelings and also gives clients permission to protect themselves from painful feelings they are not yet ready to face.

Some questions that have been used during the research process to assist clients to develop diagnostic images and which can be used clinically to help elicit feelings, dissatisfactions, tensions, or unhealthy images are:

1. Go inside yourself and locate where any feelings of anger or resentment are in your body. Tell me what you see. Anything else?
2. Where in your body are there any feelings of guilt? What are you picturing? Anything else?
3. Where in your body are there any feelings of sadness? What do you see? Anything else?
4. Now scan your body once more for any feelings or images you might have missed. Describe what you see now.

While answering these questions it is common for clients to become aware of strong feelings that were not in awareness or to learn the image of their body was misshapen or of distressing color or texture. Other clients may comment that they knew about some of the feelings or images but had not been able to integrate them into an understandable whole until using the imagery approach.

Sometimes it is useful to ask clients to picture how the feelings are affecting their muscle tension, blood flow, hormonal secretions, or general body functioning. Some clients will describe these effects spontaneously. For example, one client reported, "tightness in my breathing in my chest—I see a blue plastic band like the ones around broccoli—I want to cut it."

Preliminary research results suggest that clients do offer an entirely different order of information about their perceived health problems when asked to use Diagnostic Guided Imagery as opposed to when they are asked traditional intake questions such as, "What brought you here today?". Some comparisons may prove useful in differentiating the two types of information.

Traditional Assessment Responses

Diagnostic Guided Imagery

1. Lack of confidence in school and social situations

1. "My stomach is contracted, shrunken like a balloon, sucked in, oozing HCL and in spasm."

2. No callus formation on fractured humerus

2. "I see the ends of two broken chicken bones; the plates are screwing metal and cold, but the bone ends are jagged. I feel anger in my fist; I'd like to punch the doctor who put in the plates without asking me. My stomach is tightening like a vice, all green and prickly. Sadness in my heart; I want to cradle it with my right arm and bend my head over to take care of it."

3. Anxiety about exams

3. "My professor is writing on the board but there's nothing written there. I see a big cave with a light at the end. I'm not afraid, but I'm dwarfed by how large the chamber is. It's tedious, monotonous trip, but beautiful at the end."

4. Angina

4. "My heart is tense and fibrillating; tight, working too hard, snapping."

5. Sore back muscle

4. "The muscle is torn and ragged, redder at the ends, instead of pink. I hurt myself lifting a piece of furniture with my brother—the one I'm always angry at."

6. Stuttering

6. "My throat is moving around, never still. Trachea is huge and it sticks out, white and hard. My lungs are scared, they're too small for the space they're in."

7. Overeating

7. "There is an animal consumed in flames someplace between my stomach and throat. There are tentacles reaching into my trunk and G-I tract, downwards to my knees and up past my shoulders. It has no head or much of a body."

8. Agitated depression

8. "Tightness in my intestines, anger is tightening in my shoulders, tautness in the middle of my back, sadness in my heart; I can only see one lung, chaotic mess of tubes and blood vessels in my chest."

Healing Guided Imagery

The clinician can choose the therapeutic images for the client, ask the client, "How would the area look if it were healthy?" or the two can collaborate to develop an individualized healing image. The therapeutic images developed for the problems assessed via Diagnostic Guided Imagery were:

Diagnostic Guided Imagery Problem

1. Stomach contracted, shrunken, sucked in, oozing HCL, spasm
2. Plates metal, cold, bone ends jagged
3. Can't read professor, trip is tedious, monotonous, beautiful at end
4. Heart tense, fibrillating, working too hard, snapping
5. Torn, ragged, red muscle

6. Throat moving around; trachea huge, sticking out, hard, white; lungs too small and scared
7. Animal consumed in flames; tentacles, no head and little body

Therapeutic Image

1. Stomach full, relaxed, healthy

2. Plates are warm, soft, bone ends are connecting.

3. Reads what professor has written on board; journey becomes less tedious and monotonous

4. Heart beating nicely

5. The torn edges of the muscle are moving together, color changing to pink, anger is placed in a container and put away

6. Throat at rest, trachea smoothing and softening, lungs expanding to fill available space

7. Flames die out, the life force is gone, no center remains, the animal deflates, lies in a puddle, leaves body as waste.

8. Tightness in intestines, anger tightening shoulders and back; heart/lungs chaotic and partial	8. Loosening and widening of muscles in gut, shoulders back; standing back from body to be able to see other lung; heart and lungs are pink, expanded, orderly

Another way to form therapeutic images is to ask the client to think of images of love, peace, joy and harmony and to picture each one's effect on muscle tension, blood flow, hormonal secretion and body functioning.

Some images that can be used (or adapted) for health or stress problems in the well population include (Samuels and Samuels, 1975; Bry, 1972; Simonton and Creighton, 1978):

Health/Stress Problem	*Therapeutic Images*
1. Headache	1. Picture a hole in your head near the area of the headache; on exhalation, imagine the pain going through the hole as a color
2. Nasal or sinus congestion	2. Imagine tubes opening and draining like a sink unclogging
3. Hemorrhoids	3. Imagine the pelvis becoming warm as you picture blood flowing into it; see your anus as cool, and becoming cooler perhaps sitting in a cool, relaxing bath
4. Anger	4. Locate the place(s) in your body where you see the anger. Now choose a container of some sort. Put all the anger in the container, cover it, and put it someplace where it cannot affect you
5. Sadness or ending a relationship	5. Locate all your feelings of sadness or ending in your body that you want to get rid of. Put all the feelings in a container that is attached to a filled balloon. Let go of the container and wave goodbye to feelings, container and balloon. Fill up any emptiness that remains in your body with images of peace, love and harmony.
6. Excessive gastric secretion	6. Picture the texture and dryness of blotting paper in your stomach area; picture absorbent dryness
7. Gynecological or menstrual problems	7. Picture your pelvis warm and healthy

8. Ineffective immune system

8. Picture healthy white blood cells moving in to attack invading viruses or bacteria; see the white blood cells carrying the weakened viruses or bacteria away, out of your body

Another way to use healing guided imagery is to picture the entire body healthy, whole, and relaxed. This kind of image can be used universally, despite the symptom or problem. It is most useful as a preventive image. Clients can be asked to picture their bodies healthy, whole, and relaxed several times a day, each day. A good time to use preventive imagery is when taking a shower or bath. The water provides the relaxation and the task allows for nearly total concentration on the therapeutic image.

PROBLEM-SOLVING GUIDED IMAGERY

Imagery can be used in a number of structured ways to assist clients to solve problems.

- *The closed box* (Bry, 1978).—Picture yourself locked up in a giant wooden box with a securely tied lid. Picture what you would do to get out of that box. (This exercise can be used to help clients discover what's wrong with their lives and how to change it. As clients begin to picture how to get out of the box, new insights regarding how to change their lives will occur to them.)
- *The blue frame* (Bry, 1978).—Clearly define the problem. Place it in a blue frame. Pretend you're telling the problem to a friend and be very specific about all aspects of the problem. See the solution to the problem in a white frame. It is suggested that a client ponder the following questions prior to attempting to solve the problem:

- Do I really want to know the answer to this problem?
- Do I feel I deserve an answer to this problem?
- Am I willing to accept the solution even if it's not what I'd hoped for?

HELPING CLIENTS CONTACT THEIR INNER ADVISER

Inner dialogue is based on the idea that everyone has an intuitive aspect that knows what to do to be healthier and happier. There are a number of different ways to get in touch with this intuitive, self-healing aspect (Clark, 1981b). One way is to enter into a dialogue with an archetypal or mythical figure. The dialogue focuses on physical symptoms and what they represent and on ways to reorder one's life, thereby releasing oneself from the symptoms (Bry, 1978). The theoretical basis of this approach is that the body is the battleground for conflicting attitudes, beliefs, and ideas. Once the client dialogues about the conflict, that conflict changes form.

Dr. Irving Oyle, a proponent of this approach, helps clients deeply relax their bodies and then directs them to go to a lake in their mind's eye and wait for a figure or animal to appear to them for the purpose of dialogue. Another way to use inner dialogue is to ask a client to depict his or her inner adviser in whatever shape or form that seems right. In time, each person will visualize an adviser form that has helpful qualities. Perseverance and honesty are necessary to be successful with this approach.

Initially clients (and clinicians) may be skeptical about this approach. For this reason, some people may try it only after many other approaches have failed to bring relief. As with other approaches, the clinician needs a positive attitude to assist the client in learning and using the technique. One way for clinicians to feel more positive is to try the technique prior to using it with clients.

This technique is not meant to be a substitute for needed medical care. However, many clients have symptoms that cannot be helped by medical intervention, such as colds, pain that does not respond to medication or for which there is no organic basis, and to receive reassurance. Some examples may help to explain the use of the inner adviser.

- Beth, a young nurse, had been proclaimed cured of breast cancer following surgery. However, she did not seem to heal or to be interested in life. She described severe, continuing pain in her back, "like a tiger clawing at me." Pain medication did not help. A nurse on the unit taught Beth the inner dialogue approach. Beth learned how to relax her body and then went in search of her inner adviser. She met a tiger by a stream who told her he had been trying to get her attention by clawing at her. The tiger told Beth she had never wanted to be a nurse but had gone through nursing school to please her parents. Resentment and unfulfilled dreams had led her to cancer. The tiger told Beth to decide what she wanted to do with her life and do it and then her pain would be bearable. After several sessions of dialogue, Beth reported less pain.
- Warren is a teacher who recently bought a house with his wife. He worked every evening on the house after teaching all day. Recently he had incurred several injuries including a pulled back muscle, a sprained thumb, and a broken toe. His wife read about the inner advisor technique and asked him to try it to find out why he was getting so many injuries. Warren laughed at first, but finally agreed. With persistence he was able to contact his inner adviser, an American Indian woman who told him he was being pulled in so many directions that he was injuring himself. The inner adviser told him to slow down and not try to do so much work on the house at once and that life is to enjoy. After Warren cut his time on the house in half, he incurred no further injuries.

Before using the inner adviser approach, clients can prepare themselves by asking a series of questions:

- If I had an inner adviser, what would he, she, or it look like?
- What characteristics would my inner adviser have that would be helpful to me?
- What is the best way to communicate with my inner adviser?
- What familial body vulnerabilities might I be getting messages about? (For example, do people in my family tend to show conflict by getting colds, backaches, diarrhea, or some other symptom?)
- What are my usual body symptoms that may be giving me messages about imbalances in my body/mind?
- In what ways have I been misusing my body/mind lately?
- In what direction is my life going that I do not want it to go?

The answers to these questions provide valuable clues about what to expect and provide the beginning experience for inner dialogue. Following this preparatory stage, the client is helped to engage in a relaxation exercise.

Suggestions for consulting an inner adviser include the following:

1. Choose a time when you are not rushed. Relax your body completely using a relaxation exercise.
2. Totally focus on picturing your inner adviser. Go to a place where you are comfortable and at peace. Wait peacefully and expectantly for your inner adviser to appear.
3. Picture very clearly what your inner adviser looks like, including size, shape, age, dress.
4. Find a comfortable physical distance between you and your inner adviser.
5. Begin to communicate with your adviser. Find out what kind of an adviser you have. Ask questions about your health or life problems.
6. Realize that communication with your inner adviser may seem silly or stilted at first or that it may be perfectly natural; take whatever happens in stride. Give yourself permission to continue and to work toward optimum communication with your inner adviser.
7. When you have obtained answers to your questions, return to the here and now.
8. Allow yourself to feel good about your progress and what you have learned.
9. Make a plan for using what you learned and be confident you can change.

Inner dialogue may be of the most help to clients with psychosomatic symptoms. They are usually the least aware of the meaning of their symptoms. If they were more aware of their inner conflicts, they may not have developed the symptoms in the first place. Inner dialogue may also be of great help to clients who are unable to verbalize their thoughts and feelings directly. Clients who use self-blame or guilt may find help through inner dialogue too; it is a structured way of providing positive new direction without focusing on self-destructive feelings that may interfere with wellness.

Inner dialogue can also be used to solve problems. Nurses may turn to their inner "nursing adviser" for intuitive help with a nursing problem. Clients who want to solve a work-related problem can turn to their inner "work adviser." Inner dialogue can be carried on with aspects of the social, work, intimate, student, family, or political self. As many inner advisers as needed can be consulted about everyday or emergency situations.

REFERENCES

Bry, A. (1972). *Directing the movies of your mind*. New York: Harper & Row, pp. 131–164.

Clark, C.C. (1981a). *Enhancing wellness: A guide for self-care*. New York: Springer Publishing, pp. 4–6.

Clark, C.C. (1981b). Inner dialogue: A self-healing approach for nurses and clients. *American Journal of Nursing, 81*(6), 1191–1193.

Curtis J.D., & Detert, R.A. (1981). *How to relax: A holistic approach to stress management*. Palo Alto, CA: Mayfield Publishing, p. 148.

Davis, M., McKay, M., & Eshelman, E.R. (1980). *The relaxation and stress reduction workbook*. Richmond, CA: New Harbinger Publications, pp. 112–125.

Grinder, J., & Bandler, R. (1981). *Trance-formations, neurolinguistic programming and the structure of hypnosis*. Moab, UT: Real People Press, 14–15.

Samuels, M., & Samuels, N. (1975). *Seeing with the mind's eye*. New York: Random House, pp. 156–238.

Simonton, O.C., Simonton, S., & Creighton, J. (1978). *Getting well again*. New York: J. P. Tarcher, pp. 131–139.

PART II

Clinical Applications: Pain

6

Treatment of Pain: Theory and Research

Susan Plock Bromley

When considering the use of hypnosis in pain management, the therapist is likely to find that the client has many misconceptions and fears about both pain and hypnosis. Neither pain nor hypnosis has ever been satisfactorily understood or defined. Many myths have evolved to explain why we have pain and how hypnosis works. Patients tend to view their pain as caused by external forces, whether germs, instruments of trauma, or supernatural entities. Chronic pain sufferers frequently turn to religion to understand their pain. There are many religious explanations ranging from pain as punishment to pain as salvation (Bakan, 1968; Brena, 1972; Keele, 1957). Similarly most patients believe that hypnosis is an external, perhaps even supernatural, power of the therapist that will be used to control them. Very few believe initially that they have control both of their pain and their hypnotic state. Pain and hypnosis, then, are considered by most to be ego-dystonic and mysterious. People tend to turn to experts for help with pain and for hypnosis.

But it is not just clients who have misconceptions. Helen Neal (1978) noted that even those who don't classify themselves as religious or superstitious are influenced by pain folklore because it is passed from generation to generation not only through religious training but also through societal codes of moral and social behavior. Progress in understanding how pain works and how to control it has been impeded by centuries of folklore (Beecher, 1965), and hypnosis is underutilized as a pain control method because of widespread superstition (Crasilneck & Hall, 1975).

Given these conditions, it is essential for hypnotherapists to become aware of sources of bias about pain and hypnosis, and to be able to identify these both

The author expresses her appreciation to the University of Northern Colorado at Greeley for grant assistance with the manuscript.

in themselves and their clients. Only then can we proceed to help clients use imagery to control pain.

PAIN THEORY

For centuries three concepts of pain coexisted peacefully: pain as a bodily sensation, pain as an emotion and pain as a manifestation of supernatural forces or disharmony with nature (Dallenbach, 1939; Keele, 1957). With the development of scientific study of the body, the metaphysical concepts of pain were relegated to religion or philosophy, and controversy arose regarding the exact etiology of pain. At the beginning of the 20th century, some scientists remained convinced that pain was an emotion rather than a sensation. Others who contended that pain was neurologically based were divided by their support of either the *specificity* or the *intensity/pattern* theory of pain. The more prominent *specificity* theory proposed that pain was an independent sensation with its own transmission system and that pain intensity was related to severity of the injury or disease. The *intensity/pattern* theory proposed that sensory nerves and receptors were not specialized, but carried many different messages from the periphery to the brain. It proposed that pain messages were not tied to severity but instead occured when neural impulses exceeded a certain intensity level and/or when a certain pattern of neural messages were sent to the brain (Melzack, 1973; Hardy, Wolff, & Goodell, 1952).

Two major misconceptions arising from this era of controversy continue to complicate current pain treatment. First, pain was considered to be only a symptom of an underlying disease or trauma. Consequently research and treatment neglected pain, relegating it instead to a secondary symptom which would automatically disappear with treatment of the primary problem of disease or trauma. This approach has been successful with acute but not chronic pain problems (Bonica, 1980).

Second, pain problems were viewed as evolving from either physical *or* emotional sources instead of being comprised of both components. This dichotomous thinking, reminiscent of Descarte's concept of mind/body dualism led to major problems as experts fruitlessly attempted to differentiate between "real/organic" versus "functional/imaginary" pain (Fordyce, 1976; Merskey, 1980; Sternbach, 1978).

It wasn't until 1965 when Melzack and Wall proposed the *gate control* theory of pain that the three formerly irreconcilable pain theories were integrated. Their theory has stimulated many new avenues of research and treatment including increased acceptance of hypnosis as a legitimate pain control technique (Melzack & Wall, 1965, 1982).

Physiological Aspects

After almost 20 years of research, the basic tenets of the *gate control* theory of pain remain dominant (Melzack & Wall, 1982). This theory proposes that sensory input from the environment and from within the body is received by many specialized neural receptors throughout the body. These receptors transmit multiple messages regarding pain location and intensity via non-specialized large-diameter (A-beta) and small-diameter (A-delta and C) nerve fibers. Some messages, particularly those regarding assessment of danger in the pain situation, are sent directly to the brain via fast-conducting, large-diameter myelenated nerves. Other pain messages are sent via smaller, slower nerves to the ganglia of the sympathetic nervous system, just outside the spinal cord. Most pain messages are believed to be coordinated in the substantial gelatinosa of the spinal cord and controlled by transmission (T) cells in the dorsal horn of the spinal cord. These T cells contain a "pain gating" mechanism. When pain is of sufficient intensity, the gate opens, sending pain messages to the brain, where they are interpreted. When the gate is closed no messages of pain are sent to the brain. Prior to reaching the T cells, pain information is modulated by interaction between the large-diameter nerve fibers, which tend to inhibit pain messages, and the small-diameter nerve fibers, which transmit them. Other nerve cells in areas like the substantial gelatinosa in the spinal cord or the sympathetic ganglia just outside the spinal cord may also modulate pain messages prior to their reaching the T cells. Pain messages may be further modified by neural input further up the spinal cord as well as by neural messages descending from the brain.

In addition T cells may transmit pain messages via two different neural systems in the spinal cord to two major brain areas (Melzack & Wall, 1982). One system seems to be involved in the transmission of the sensory and discriminative dimensions of pain-like intensity and type of pain. This kind of information is believed to be transmitted via neospinothalamic fibers to the brain's ventrobasal thalamus and somatosensory cortex. The other system seems to be involved with the unpleasant emotions and motivation that trigger pain responses. These messages are thought to be transmitted by medially coursing nerve fibers into the reticular formation, medial and intralaminar thalamus, and limbic system areas of the brain.

Melzack and Wall hypothesized that a system in the neocortex evaluates input from these two systems along with stored pain information such as memory of past experiences. At the same time the brain is receiving other relevant information, such as the degree of danger in the situation and the availability of help. Almost simultaneously, the brain sends messages back down the spinal cord based on the integrated interpretation of events. These descending messages further modify the T cell transmission of pain messages. The psychological components of the brain's descending messages seem to be more important than had initially been expected in modifying pain perception (Melzack & Wall, 1982).

The incredible complexity of this process indicates why it has been impossible thus far to adequately define and treat pain. At the same time, it becomes clear why researchers have found that pain relief is often only achieved by multiple treatment modalities. Theorists now contend that different physiological and psychological pain treatment techniques affect different neural messages (Hilgard & Hilgard, 1975; Melzack & Wall, 1982; Sternbach, 1978).

Consequently, current practice, particularly in pain treatment centers, is to use multiple, concurrent treatment techniques in an effort to find the specific successful combination for each sufferer (Melzack & Wall, 1982; Sternbach, 1974).

Biochemical Aspects

Neurotransmitters send messages along the nerves. The kind of chemical present in the neural path and its concentration affect the type and intensity of the message. Certain chemicals manufactured by the body, such as bradykinin, are known to cause pain. It is common knowledge that drugs of the opium family are transmitted across neurons and inhibit pain. In 1977 researchers found that the body itself produced analgesic chemicals: endorphins and enkaphalins (Snyder, 1980; Terenius, 1979; West, 1981). Melzack and Wall (1982), reviewing several studies, concluded that endorphins and enkaphalins seem to exert some continuous inhibition of pain. They may also be released in highly concentrated amounts during arousal of the autonomic nervous system, to protect the individual from overwhelming pain.

Concentrations of endorphins and enkaphalins occur both in the brain and in the spinal cord. Special opoid receptors have been found in neurons in these areas. But in some neural areas, opoid receptors exist with no concentration of enkaphalins and endorphins, and vice versa, which indicates that research has not unraveled all the mysteries of these chemicals (Hunt, Kelly, & Emerson, 1980).

Endorphins and enkaphalins are believed to work like opiate drugs, because their action is blocked by naloxone, a morphine antagonist. However, naloxone does not block analgesia of certain pain stimuli, which indicates that other, non-opoid chemicals in the body, might also be serving as natural analgesics (Dennis & Melzack, 1980; Lindblom & Tegner, 1979). Some other biochemicals believed to be involved in natural analgesia are noradrenalin, acetylcholine, and dopamine (Melzack & Wall, 1982). Interestingly, pain relief due to placebos is blocked by naloxone, but hypnotic analgesia *is not* interrupted by naloxone (Goldstein & Hilgard, 1975; Hilgard, 1980). This suggests that the placebo effect and hypnotic analgesia involve different biochemical and neural aspects of the body's pain control system.

It is also hypothesized that with chronic pain, as with some depressions, slow but long-acting biochemical changes might contribute to maintenance of pain after the initial cause has been treated successfully. The apparent similarity between the two conditions may be even more widespread than is now suspected, because tricyclic antidepressants relieve both some kinds of depression and some kinds of chronic pain (Melzack & Wall, 1982; Sternbach, 1974).

Psychological Aspects

The gate control theory has provided the link between the physiological and psychological factors in pain through recognition of the powerful modulating force of the brain's descending messages on pain perception. Psychological factors are now believed to be so central to pain control that pain experts are defining pain as a primarily psychological event rather than a purely physical sensation (Bonica, 1980; Iasp., 1979; NINCDS, 1979). Certain psychological factors seem to be consistently related to the pain experience. "Psychological" refers to mental processes including learning, memory, emotions, perception, and personality characteristics, as well as environmental interactions including social and cultural factors (Jacox, 1977).

Past Experience and Learning

Acknowledgment that pain is both instinctive and learned has led to many hypotheses and discoveries (Weisenberg, 1977b). Chapman (1978), in reviewing perceptual pain theory, noted that as we mature we develop a body concept as a whole or "gestalt." He hypothesized that phantom limb pain may occur because of the discrepancy between our internalized percept of our whole body and the new, nonintegrated fact of a missing limb. Szasz (1957), proposes that we develop object relations with our body as we do with other people and concludes that pain gives rise to the same kind of fears of loss that we experience in our relationships with others.

Implicit in the concept of learned pain is the fact that we remember recurrent painful experiences. Memory of past painful events significantly influences our perception of current painful situations. This is particularly evident in people who must repeatedly endure painful procedures, like burn victims. These patients, who must deal daily with painful dressing changes and debridement procedures, begin to experience pain and anxiety prior to the procedure, which intensifies the pain of the actual procedure.

Theorists concur that multiple or severely painful childhood experiences predispose adults to chronic pain conditions (Engel, 1959; Fordyce, 1976; Merskey & Spear, 1967; Pilowski, 1978).

Language, which is learned, also seems to shape the pain experience. Words help us communicate the nature of pain (Melzack, 1975; Merskey, 1972); words also become conditioned stimuli that both elicit and inhibit pain, as evidenced by the power of chants and prayers (Frank, 1961; Keele, 1957).

Meaning and Context of the Pain Experience

We know that a skinned knee sustained during a tennis game does not seem to hurt nearly as badly as a skinned knee sustained on the way to an important meeting. Beecher's studies of military and civilian wounded emphasizes the importance of the pain context (Beecher, 1959). When Zahourek and I conducted an informal burn study at Denver General Hospital, we encountered a striking example of this phenomena. A 54-year-old woman had been burned on about 30 percent of her body. She experienced good pain relief with both hypnosis and drugs; however, *nothing* could contain her pain between 11:00 A.M. and 1:00 P.M. Numerous drug combinations; alternating times of her lunch, debridement, and dressing change; and hypnosis were all unsuccessful. In discussion with her, we discovered that the fire had occurred during these hours and she felt guilty about not having been able to prevent injury to one of the children for whom she was babysitting. After being encouraged to talk about her guilt, she finally achieved pain relief during these hours.

Not only the circumstances surrounding painful experiences but also the severity and prognosis of the illness or injury have profound effects on the experience of pain. Terminal illness, the loss of a limb, or permanent loss of functioning all exacerbate pain perception; a transitory injury like a sprained ankle will hurt, but the pain will not be intensified by the fear and anxiety that accompany more permanent and disabling conditions (Sacerdote, 1980; Sternbach, 1968).

Emotions

Perhaps the most widely documented finding in both clinical and experimental research is the association of anxiety with acute pain conditions (Pelletier, 1977). Reduction of anxiety usually leads to pain reduction. Sternbach (1968) noted that the anxiety and acute pain states are similar physiologically; both produce a state of autonomic arousal. McCaffery (1972) emphasized the necessity of determining the source of anxiety. A patient may be experiencing intense pain exacerbated by anxiety unrelated to the illness or injury. A 27-year-old participant in the burn study conducted at the Denver General Hospital responded well but inconsistently to hypnosis for pain relief. In exploring his personal situation, we found that there were some unresolved marital and family problems which surfaced at different times during his hospitalization. When his family problems increased, his pain relief decreased. Utilization of therapy in addition to hypnosis helped him deal more effectively with both his pain and family problems.

Personality/Psychiatric Disorders

The underlying assumption of psychosomatic medicine was that certain personality types are prone to specific physical disorders, and that the personality had to be treated to cure the disease. The literature describes the "migraine personality" (Harrison, 1975), the "low pack pain personality" (Leavitt, 1982), the "pain prone personality" (Engel, 1959); the "painful person" (Szasz, 1974), and many others. Others insist that several personality types, rather than one, are associated with chronic pain (Hendler, 1981; Sternbach, 1974). Some common personality traits have been identified in chronic illness and pain sufferers (Pilowsky & Spence, 1976). No specific personality characteristics, however, clearly distinguish one chronic disease from another.

More at issue is whether chronic pain precipitates personality changes or whether certain personality characteristics precipitate painful conditions. Evidence exists that both situations occur. Some people have mental disturbances that disappear with the alleviation of pain. Others have backgrounds and/or mental disorders that predispose them to having chronic pain as a symptom (Engel, 1959; Fordyce, 1976; Hendler, 1981; Pilowski, 1978; Szasz, 1974; Sternbach, 1974).

Merskey and Spear (1967) extensively reviewed the literature and conducted studies to determine how and when pain occurs as a symptom in psychiatric disorders. They found that pain was a frequent symptom in depression, anxiety states, and hysterical personality disorders. Pain was less prominent in obsessive-compulsive disorders, organic confusional states, and antisocial personality disorders. Merskey (1972, 1978) proposed that three types of painful conditions are caused by primarily psychological mechanisms: (1) pain as an hallucination in association with schizophrenia or psychotic depression (rare); (2) pain due to stress-induced muscle tension or vascular distention resulting in, for instance, tension or migraine headaches; and (3) conversion disorders, in which pain occurs as a result of psychological events.

In summary, chronic pain seems to trigger psychological responses such as depression, anger, and withdrawal; certain persons whose lives have been marked by pain and unhappiness may be predisposed to having chronic pain; some psychiatric disorders like conversion hysteria have pain as a prominent symptom; and some pain may be precipitated by psychologically based problems like stress. It is unlikely that researchers will find a one-to-one relationship between specific personality types and specific chronic pain problems.

Environmental Factors and Operant Behavior

Fordyce (1976) proposed that all behavior reflecting the presence of pain, including speech, facial expression, posture, taking medications, seeking health care and refusing to exercise or work, originated with the painful stimulus in acute pain situations. With chronic pain, these behaviors may remain due to environmental reinforcement, such as escape from a disliked job. Soon, the pain response occurs to *elicit* the environmental reward, not because of a preceeding noxious stimulus. This kind of pain Fordyce refers to as "operant" pain. Possible environmental reinforcers may include "as needed" pain medications, overprotective or oversolicitous family, and workmen's compensation; to extinguish this behavior one has to remove the environmental contingencies that reward pain behavior.

Other environmental interactions seem to affect pain intensity such as peer group pressure, persons near you at the time of pain, (Craig & Weiss, 1971), family attitudes (Gentry, Shaw, & Thomas, 1974; Johnson & Baldwin, 1968), family size (Gonda, 1962; Merskey & Spear, 1967), and birth order (Collins & Stone, 1966). Others have found that ethnic and cultural identification influences how one experiences and expresses pain to others (Weisenberg, 1977a; Wolff & Langley, 1968; Zbrowski, 1969; Zola, 1966).

Coping Techinques

Controlling the painful situation, getting appropriate information, and distraction all seem to diminish pain. The more one perceives control over the painful situation, the higher the pain tolerance (Bowers, 1971; Staub, Tursky & Schwartz, 1971). Instructions and information affect the amount of experimental pain a person will tolerate (Blitz & Dinnerstein, 1968; Bobey & Davidson, 1970), and the degree of postsurgical pain (Gaines, Smith & Skolnick, 1977). Natural childbirth incorporates education, which helps reduce labor pain (Davenport & Boylon, 1974). Knowledge in general affects pain perception, but the type of information given, the timing, the patient's anxiety level, personality characteristics, and other variables interact in such a complex manner that it is difficult to predict the sole influence of information on pain perception.

PAIN CONTROL METHODS

Hypnosis is just one of many techniques used in pain control, and in itself is not helpful for everyone nor for every kind of pain. For chronic pain, particularly, two or more methods of pain control used concurrently may be more successful than a single method. Physical methods of pain control include chemical analgesia and anesthesia (Gebhart, 1977; Melzack & Wall, 1982; Sternbach, 1974; Twycross, 1978), surgery (Hilgard & Hilgard, 1975; Melzack & Wall, 1982; McDonnel, 1977), acupuncture (Armstrong, 1977; Melzack & Wall, 1982; Lewitt, 1979; Hilgard, 1980; Ghia, Mao, Toomey & Gregg, 1976), and electrical stimulation (Melzack & Wall, 1982).

Psychological Methods

More psychological pain control methods are currently being used, particularly in pain treatment centers. In addition to hypnosis, the most frequently used are biofeedback, behavior therapy, relaxation techniques, and traditional psychotherapy.

Biofeedback

Biofeedback is a psychophysiological method that facilitates voluntary control over physiological processes. In this procedure a person is attached to a machine by electrodes or sensors. The machine amplifies physiological processes such as muscle tension, blood flow, temperature, or brain waves, translating the physiological activity into auditory or visual signals. By learning to modify a tone or light, the patient learns to control physiological responses. Biofeedback has been particularly successful in helping patients control both tension and migraine headaches (Budzynski, 1977; Budzynski et al., 1973; Greenspan, 1981).

There is controversy regarding the relationship between hypnosis and biofeedback. Both methods involve cognitive regulation of autonomic functions, and both employ distraction. However, hypnotic techniques stress modes of pain denial, whereas biofeedback emphasizes the development of sensitivity to bodily processes (Elton, Burrows, & Stanley, 1980; Hilgard,

1980). Some evidence indicates that a good hypnosis candidate may not be a good candidate for biofeedback, and vice versa (Hilgard, 1980). Another study found that there was no difference between high and low hypnotizables and their successful use of biofeedback (Holroyd et al., 1979). Transfer of training from clinic to home seems to be more easily accomplished with hypnosis than biofeedback (Elton et al., 1980).

Behavior Therapy

Behavior therapy is particularly successful in the treatment of chronic pain conditions that involve operant pain behavior maintained by environmental contingencies (Sternbach, 1974; Fordyce, 1976, 1978, 1980). The focus with operant conditioning is on living with pain more successfully by changing environmental contingencies.

Hypnosis is often combined with behavior therapy to achieve pain reduction. Kroger and Fezler (1976) have developed an extensive system of combining these two methods. They, along with others, believe that hypnotic inductions strengthen behavior techniques (Dempsey & Granich, 1978; Dengrove, 1976; Lazarus, 1973; Weitzenhoffer, 1972). However, Wadden and Anderton (1982), in a literature review, concluded that hypnotic induction does not enhance behavioral techniques.

Relaxation Techinques

The many forms of relaxation therapy, such as transcendental meditation, progressive relaxation (Jacobson, 1938), and the relaxation response (Benson, 1975), seem to diminish discomfort by eliciting the parasympathetic nervous system response. These techniques are used with biofeedback, behavior therapy, and hypnosis to enhance pain control.

There has been controversy about the relative effectiveness of meditation versus hypnosis. Hilgard (1980) noted that the discrepancies in the effectiveness of the two techniques disappear when adjustment is made for duration of treatment; most studies of physiological changes accomplished through meditation are based on longterm treatment, whereas results of hypnosis are usually measured after very few, or even one, session.

Hypnosis seems to be more than just another form of relaxation. Although relaxation techniques are used in hypnosis, hypnotic induction does not require relaxation (Hilgard, 1980). And hypnotic analgesia has been found to produce more pain relief than relaxation alone (Hilgard & Hilgard, 1975).

Psychotherapy

Psychotherapy is most certainly indicated when pain problems seem to be associated with underlying mental disorders (Merskey & Spear, 1967; Pilowski, 1978; Sternbach, 1974). In addition to individual therapy, group and family therapy have been successfully used with many chronic pain patients (Fordyce, 1976; Hendler, 1981). Hypnosis in conjunction with psychodynamic or behavior therapy has been successfully used with patients in pain (Fromm & Schor, 1972; Kroger & Fezler, 1976). Ego-strengthening hypnotic techniques are used extensively to increase self-esteem and decrease chronic pain (Crasilneck & Hall, 1975; Elton et al., 1980; Hartland, 1971).

HYPNOSIS

Current Status

Debate continues regarding the mechanism by which hypnosis aids in pain reduction. The traditional assumption has been that hypnosis results in an altered state of consciousness (Fromm & Shor, 1972; Hartland, 1971; Needham and Outterson-Wood, 1955). Others contend that hypnosis does not involve a special departure from normal consciousness and does not require trance induction (Barber, 1977; Sarbin & Slagle, 1980). Orne (1980) stressed that it is the context in which hypnosis is used that determines subjects' compliance, thus dismissing this controversy as irrelevant. Hilgard (1980) proposed an interesting and perhaps more helpful variation in this controversy with his dissociation theory. He found that hypnosis involves "cognitive control changes" rather than changes in the quality of consciousness. In his experimental pain studies, Hilgard has shown that subjects seem to demonstrate two separate ego functions—a hypnotized part of the self who reports minimal pain and an observing part that acknowledges accurate pain perception. The hypnotized part of the self seems to be unaware of the "hidden observer," thus presenting a dissociative phenomenon (Hilgard & Hilgard, 1975).

The other major debate revolves around the relationship between hypnotic susceptibility and pain control. People vary in their responsiveness to hypnosis. Generally it is believed that approximately 10 percent of the population is nonsusceptible, 30 percent achieve a light state, 30 percent a moderate state, and the other 30 percent are deeply hypnotizable. Although a person may achieve some increased depth over time, this change seems to be minimal.

While clinicians tend to minimize the need to determine degree of hypnotizibility when using hypnosis for pain relief (Sacerdote, 1980), clinical and experimental researchers contend that degree of hypnotizibility does affect the amount of pain relief achieved (Karlin & Morgan, 1979). Hilgard (1980) has found that people of low hypnotizibility can achieve about 20 per cent pain reduction but that highly susceptible subjects achieve significantly more pain relief. Wadden and Anderton (1982) in a review of the literature, concluded that hypnotic susceptibility is a major factor in the amount of pain relief achieved and criticize clinicians and researchers for their failure to consider susceptibility levels as a major variable in their studies.

In spite of controversy regarding exactly how hypnosis leads to diminished discomfort, there is consensus that hypnosis is an effective method of pain control. Most specialists also agree that it is not just hypnotizibility which varies in individuals but also their interests, motives, and capabilities. Many believe that those factors as well as the quality of the client–hypnotist relationship are equally important in determining pain relief (Crasilneck, 1980; Hilgard, 1980; Zahourek, 1982). Consequently, hypnotists need to determine what kind of induction and instructions best fit the specific needs of their clients. For instance, some patients may respond best to suggestions of visual imagery, while others respond better to suggestions involving bodily distortion or even auditory and olfactory hallucinations. Although the current trend is toward permissive techniques with suggestions of self-control and self-mastery, some patients find more authoritarian techniques effective. Even people who are not susceptible to hypnosis can achieve relaxation and decrease anxiety through the use of imagery and suggestion (Hilgard, 1980). Nurses find when a patient is not in a trance state, relaxation, distraction, and imagery techniques produce increased comfort (McCaffery, 1972; 1980; 1981; Rodger, 1972).

Patient motivation is crucial (Crasilneck, 1980). At Denver General Hospital, we found that some patients achieved trance state successfully when experiencing pain, but lost their ability as they healed. Just as important is the hypnotist's motivation. It was found that if the professional doubted the efficacy of hypnosis or was attempting to induce hypnosis in order not to have to deal with the patient's complaints, patients were neither able to be hypnotized nor to achieve pain relief.

Direct Methods

Within the numerous variations there are some general hypnotic techniques for diminishing discomfort. The most straightforward is a direct suggestion of pain reduction. There has been a myth that the word "pain" should not be used in such a suggestion because it might exacerbate the painful sensation. However, there seems to be little factual corroboration for this concern (Hilgard, 1980). It is important, though, not to suggest that the pain will disappear completely. This invites failure and is liable to discourage the patient from using hypnosis. It is better to suggest that the pain will lessen and may not even be felt. Semiscientific or neurophysiological metaphors might help the patient focus on how to control pain. For instance, one might suggest that the patient switch off or dim nerve currents as one does with electric currents in lights to switch off or diminish the pain.

Another direct technique is the suggestion of analgesia to the painful site, such as "Your broken arm will feel numb as if it were full of novacaine." Elton et al. (1980) reported an interesting use of this technique with a chronic pain patient who had multiple pain problems—low back pain, hip pain radiating down his legs, chest muscle spasms, headache, neck pain, and limited head rotation—as a result of two serious car accidents and multiple surgical procedures. He had undergone many surgical procedures for pain relief, had tried several pain pills and even acupuncture to no avail. He was hypnotizable but did not respond to direct suggestions of pain relief. So they gave him a technical article on endorphins and enkaphalins sufficiently complicated so that he believed it was "real." They then induced hypnosis by the arm levitation method and suggested that when his arm levitated it would trigger endorphins 15 times stronger than morphine to spill into his body to give him relief. This imagery was successful for everything but his neck. The clinicans then suggested that another vial of endorphins and joint lubricants would be released in his body with the levitation of his other hand. Each time he needed the double suggestion, but was finally able to achieve pain relief.

Transfer Methods

A variation on suggestion of anaesthesia is the transference of numbness from a nonpainful site such as the hand to another area of the body; this is sometimes called the "glove anaesthesia technique." It has been found that it is easier to imagine numbness in an extremity, particularly if it isn't painful. The hypnotherapist then suggests that the numb hand rub the painful site to anesthetize it. This technique has also been used to anesthesize areas prior to painful procedures, such as the jaw for dentistry and the stomach for labor and delivery (See Chapter 9). Some patients might argue this is nonsensical, but the hypnotist can point out that the hand is already numb and so the concept of numbness in another part of the body is logical. Hilgard (1980) found substitution numbness for pain works well for moderate hypnotizables, while transfer of numbness is better achieved by the highly hypnotizable.

With chronic pain patients, displacement or alteration of pain symptoms seems to be most useful. For unknown reasons it seems that pain is more tolerable in the extremities. Perhaps we are more used to injuries to extremities like cuts and bruises and this pain is less often life threatening than pain in the more central areas. With the displacement technique, one can suggest that pain be transferred to an extremity. Many cases are reported in the literature using this technique. One of the most interesting is Erickson's (1967) account of a man dying of extremely painful cancer of the prostate. Erickson suggested that the patient transfer this pain to his left hand. The patient then became accustomed to the pain in his left hand and felt no more bodily pain. Sacerdote (1970) reported a similar case in which a patient was able to transfer his abdominal cancer pain to his left little finger.

A related concept is that of transferring the pain source from internal to external. McCaffery (1972) discussed the technique of externalizing pain, citing the example of a migraine sufferer putting her fingers on her head and imagining the pressure to be coming from her fingers instead of inside her head. McCaffery explained that when patients can externalize their pain source their anxiety tends to decrease, as they are less afraid of their own bodies being out of control.

Another technique useful in chronic pain involves the alteration rather than displacement of pain sensation. In one instance, I assisted a patient with phantom limb pain to change the pain sensation to a tingling. Another patient learned to experience his low back pain as a sense of pressure. Zahourek reported that some of her patients are able to translate their pain into color, which varies in intensity and hue as the pain fluctuates (private conversation, 1984). The advantage of these techniques for chronic pain is that patients can continue to monitor fluctuation in pain intensity even when the pain is displaced or the pain sensation is modified.

Dissociative Methods

Hypnosis may also be utilized to help patients remove themselves completely from their painful situations. Some are able to regress to a happy time prior to their painful condition. Others are able to "remove" themselves in the present time to a nonpainful place. Erickson (1976) wrote of a woman with chronic pain who learned self-hypnosis and could, when in trance, go into the living room in her wheelchair to watch TV, leaving her suffering body behind in the bedroom.

One of my patients developed a creative variation of the technique of removal of self from the painful situation. His case also demonstrates vividly the necessity of consulting with patients regarding the most helpful imagery for them. John suffered from a chronic knee injury which he frequently reinjured, with accompanying pain and swelling. He agreed to use hypnosis for both pain and fluid reduction. While he was hypnotized, I suggested that the discomfort would diminish and the fluid would be carried back up his leg to his kidneys and then expelled through his urine. His thighs then began to redden and swell. I brought him out of the trance and asked about the imagery. He was not scientifically oriented and felt that this image would cause swelling of the rest of his leg. When asked what image might be better for him, he suggested that he imagine unhooking his leg at the knee and hanging the lower leg upside down to drain on a phone line outside the window. He returned to a hypnotic state and this suggestion was given. He then achieved both pain relief and reduction of swelling in his knee.

There are many variations of all of these techniques; the most creative suggestions will often come from your clients. In addition to suggestions while in trance, many have found that the development of a key word associated with peace is helpful when returning to the trance state using self-hypnosis. Elton et al. (1980) mentioned that one woman used the word "snow" to return to the state of relaxation because it signified to her a pure, cool, lovely state. A client of mine chose to use the Spanish word for butterfly, which signified peace and freedom for him.

Hypnosis Applied To Painful Conditions

Hypnosis has been used most extensively in the management of acute pain. Application of hypnosis to chronic pain states has appeared more recently in the literature. Dentists have used hypnosis for pain, gagging, blood and saliva control, and dental phobias, with case reports published as early as 1837. Chronic pain victims suffering from temporomandibular joint syndrome are also being treated with hypnosis by dentists (Barber, 1977; Gerschman, Reade, & Burrows, 1980; Hartland, 1971; Hilgard, 1980). As discussed in Chapters 8 and 9 of this book, hypnosis has been used to control pain due to surgery and labor and delivery. The other major use of hypnosis in acute care has been with burn victims, to help with pain, appetite, healing rate, and control of infection (Ewin, 1979; Hilgard, 1980; Schafer, 1975; Wadden & Anderton, 1982). Chronic pain conditions which have been helped by hypnosis include cancer (*American Journal of Clinical Hypnosis*, 1983; Pettit, 1979; Sacerdote, 1980), headaches (Cedercreutz, 1978; Wadden & Anderton, 1982), multiple pain (Elton et al., 1980), Raynaud's disease (Braun, 1979), and phantom limb pain (Cedercreutz & Uusitalo, 1967; Hilgard, 1980).

ASSESSMENT FOR INTERVENTION AND OUTCOME

There are several variables to consider when assessing the use of hypnosis for pain management. One needs to assess the nature and extent of the pain, the personality of the person in pain, hypnotizability, what techniques should be used, and suitable outcome measures.

Assessment and Outcome Measurement

Pain assessment includes several variables such as onset, location, duration, intensity, and quality. Johnson (1977), Melzack (1975), McCaffery (1972), and McGuire (1981) have all devised helpful guidelines for comprehensively assessing the multiple aspects of pain.

After a comprehensive pain assessment, the clinician may want to measure change in pain due to intervention by shorter procedures. There are several measurement scales available ranging from simple Likert scales (Stewart, 1977) to the more extensive McGill Pain Questionnaire (Melzack, 1975) which utilizes 20 groups of words that describe pain. This questionnaire, although still a research instrument, is proving to be quite valuable in differentiating how various interventions reduce various types of pain. Other measures of pain variation are change in consumption of pain-relieving drugs or change in frequency of pain complaints. All of these methods are currently used to measure treatment outcome.

Individual Assessment

It is equally important to assess the psychological and environmental variables that may be maintaining or exacerbating the patient's pain perception. Fordyce (1976) explained how to assess environmental variables. Other assessment guidelines include psychological and social factors, which are important to consider when treating pain victims (Cummings, 1981; Johnson, 1977; Melzack, 1975; McCaffery, 1972). Certain personality tests are also used to assess pain victims, such as the Minnesota Multiphasic Personality Inventory (Sternbach, 1974) and the Illness Behavior Questionnaire (Pilowski & Spence, 1976).

Hypnosis Assessment

There are two aspects relevant to the assessment of the patient with regard to hypnotic treatment: susceptibility and technique selection. There is sufficient indication in the literature that degree of hypnotizability affects treatment outcome to merit the use of some form of rating scale to determine each person's depth of trance (Hilgard, 1980; Wadden & Anderton, 1982). Horne and Powlett (1980) have reviewed the numerous rating or susceptibility scales, which take from 15 minutes to over an hour to administer. These scales include the performance of such tasks as age regression, sensory hallucinations, posthypnotic amnesia, physical analgesia, and arm levitation. In administering one of these scales, the clinician can get an idea of what kind of technique might be most helpful for the patient to use for pain reduction, the tasks are representative of many techniques from use of imagery to use of physiological or time distortion. Although many clinicians resist the use of these scales, they are helpful assessment tools and are mandatory if conducting respectable clinical research.

CONCLUSION

Hypnosis is one tool for helping people who experience various kinds and degrees of pain. Many techniques exist and are described in other chapters in the book. It must be emphasized that these techniques are utilized within the therapeutic nursing process and are implemented from a basic understanding of both pain and hypnosis.

REFERENCES

American Journal of Clinical Hypnosis (1983). Special issue: Hypnosis and cancer, 25 (3).

Armstrong, M. E. (1977). Acupuncture. In Jacox, A. (Ed.), *Pain: A source book for nurses and other health professionals*. Boston: Little Brown, pp. 209–226.

Bakan, D. (1968) *Disease, pain and sacrifice: Toward a psychology of suffering*. Chicago: Beacon Press.

Barber, J. (1977). Rapid induction analgesics: A clinical report. *American Journal of Clinical Hypnosis, 19,* 138–147.

Beecher, H.K. (1959). *Measurement of subjective responses: Quantitative effects of drugs*. New York: Oxford University Press.

Beecher, H.K. (1965). Quantification of the subjective pain experience. In Hock, P.H., & Zubin, J. (Eds.), *Psychopathology of perception*. New York: Grune & Stratton.

Benson, H. (1975).*The relaxation response*. New York: William Morrow.

Blitz, B., & Dinnerstein, J. (1968). Effects of different types of instruction on pain parameters. *Journal of Abnormal Psychology, 73,* 276–280.

Bobey, M.J., & Davidson, P.O. (1970). Psychological factors affecting pain tolerance. *Journal of Psychosomatic Research, 14,* 371–376.

Bonica, J.J. (1980). Pain research and therapy: Past and current status and future needs. In Ng, L.K.Y., & Bonica J.J. (Eds.), *Pain, discomfort and humanitarian care*. New York: Elsevier/North Holland, Inc., 1980.

Bowers, K.S. (1971). The effects of ucs temporal uncertainty on heart rate and pain. *Psychophysiology, 8,* 382–389.

Braun, B.G. (1979). Hypnotherapy and Raynaud's disease. In Burrows, G.D., Collison, D.R., & Dennerstein, L. (Eds.), *Hypnosis 1979*. Amsterdam: Elsevier/North Holland, pp. 141–148.

Brena, S. (1972). *Pain and religion: A psychophysiological study*. Springfield, IL: Charles C. Thomas.

Budzinski, T.H. (1977). Biofeedback procedures in the clinic. In Jacox, A. (Ed.), *Pain: A source book for nurses and other health professionals*. Boston: Little Brown, 285–294.

Budzinski, T.H., Stoyva, J.M., Adler, C.S., & Mullaney, D.M. (1973). EMG biofeedback and tension headache: A controlled outcome study. *Psychosomatic Medicine, 35,* 484–496.

Cedercreutz, C. (1978). Hypnotic treatment of 100 cases of migraine. In Frankel, F.H., & Zamansky, H.S. (Eds.) 1978. *Hypnosis at its bicentennial*. New York: Plenum Press.

Cedercreutz, C., & Uusitalo, E. (1967). Hypnotic treatment of phantom sensations in 37 amputees. In Lassner J. (Ed.), *Hypnosis and psychosomatic medicine*. New York: Springer-Verlag, pp. 65–66.

Chapman, C.R. (1978). Pain: The perception of noxious events. In Sternbach, R.A. (Ed.), *The psychology of pain*. New York: Raven Press, 169–202.

Collins, L.G., & Stone, L.A. (1966). Pain sensitivity, age and activity levels in chronic schizophrenics and in normals. *British Journal of Psychiatry, 112,* 33–35.

Craig, K.D., & Weiss, S.M. (1971). Vicarious influences on pain threshold determinations. *Journal of Personality and Social Psychology, 19,* 53–59.

Crasilneck, H. (1980). Clinical assessment and preparation of the patient. In Burrows, G.D., & Dennerstein, L. (Eds.), *Handbook of hypnosis and psychosomatic medicine*. Amsterdam: Elsevier/North Holland, pp. 105–118.

Crasilneck, H.B., & Hall, J.A. (1975). *Clinical hypnosis: principles and applications*. New York: Grune & Stratton.

Cummings, D. (1981). Stopping chronic pain before it starts. *Nursing, 1,* 60–62.

Dallenbach, K.M. (1939). Pain: History and present status. *American Journal of Psychology, 52,* 331–347.

Davenport, S., & Boylon, C.A. (1974). Psychological correlates of childbirth pain. *Psychosomatic Medicine, 36,* 215–222.

Dempsey, G.L., & Granich, M. (1978). Hypno-behavioral therapy in the case of a traumatic stutter: A case study. *International Journal of Clinical and Experimental Hypnosis, 26,* 125–133.

Dengrove, E. (Ed.) (1976). *Hypnosis and behavior therapy.* Springfield, IL: Charles C. Thomas.

Dennis, S.G., & Melzack, R. (1980). Pain modulation by 5-hydroxytryptaminergic agents and morphine as measured by three pain tests. *Experimental Neurology, 69,* 260–270.

Elton, D., Burrows, G.D., & Stanley, G.V. (1980). Chronic pain and hypnosis. In Burrows, G.D. & Dennerstein, L. (Eds.), *Handbook of hypnosis and psychosomatic medicine.* Amsterdam: Elsevier/North Holland, 269–292.

Engel, G.L. (1959). Psychogenic pain and the pain-prone patient. *American Journal of Medicine, 26,* 899–918.

Engel, G.L. (1977). The need for a new medical model: A challenge for biomedicine. *Science, 196*(4286), 129–135.

Erickson, M.H. (1967). An introduction to the study and application of hypnosis for pain control. In Lassner, J. (Ed.), *Hypnosis and psychosomatic medicine.* New York: Springer-Verlag, 83–90.

Erickson, M.H. (1976). *Hypnotic realities: The induction of clinical hypnosis and forms of indirect suggestion.* New York: Irvington.

Ewin, D.M. (1979). Hypnosis in burn therapy. In Burrows, G.D., Collison, D.R. & Dennerstein, L. (Eds.) (1979). *Hypnosis 1979.* Amsterdam: Elsevier/North Holland, pp. 269–275.

Fordyce, W.E. (1976). *Behaviorial methods for chronic pain and illness.* St. Louis: C. V. Mosby.

Fordyce, W.E. (1978). Learning processes in pain. In Sternbach, R. A. (Ed.), *The psychology of pain.* New York: Raven Press, pp. 49–72.

Fordyce, W.E. (1980). A behavioral perspective on chronic pain. In Ng, L.K.Y., & Bonica J.J. (Eds.), *Pain, discomfort and humanitarian care.* New York: Elsevier/North Holland, pp. 233–252.

Frank, J.D. (1961). *Persuasion and healing.* Baltimore: Johns Hopkins Press.

Fromm, E. & Shor, R.E. (Eds.) (1972). *Hypnosis: Research developments and perspectives,* Chicago: Aldine-Atherton.

Gaines, L.S., Smith, B.D., & Skolnick, B.E. (1977), Psychological differentiation, event uncertainty, and heart rate. *Journal of Human Stress, 3*(3), 11–25.

Gebhart, G. (1977). Narcotic and nonnarcotic analgesics for relief of pain. In Jacox, A. (Ed.), *Pain: A source book for nurses and other professionals..* Boston: Little Brown, pp. 257–262.

Gentry, W.D., Shaw, W.D., & Thomas, M. (1974). Effects of modeling on pain. *Psychosomatica, 15,* 174–177.

Gerschman, J.A., Reade, P.C., & Burrows, G.D. (1980). Hypnosis and dentistry. In Burrows, G.D., & Dennerstein, L. (Eds.) *Handbook of hypnosis and psychosomatic medicine.* Amsterdam: Elsevier/North Holland, pp. 443–479.

Ghia, J.N., Mao, W., Toomey, T.C., & Gregg, J.M. (1976). Acupuncture and chronic pain mechanisms. *Pain, 2,* 285–299.

Goldstein, A., & Hilgard, E.R. (1975). Lack of influence of the morphine antagonist naloxone on hypnotic analgesia. *Proceedings of the National Academy of Sciences, 72,* 2041–2043.

Gonda, T.A. (1962). The relation between complaints of persistent pain and family size. *Journal of Neurology, Neurosurgery, and Psychiatry, 25,* 277–281.

Greenspan, K. (1981). Biofeedback in the control of chronic pain. In Mark, L.C. (Ed.), *Pain control: Practical aspects of patient care.* New York: Masson, 75–82.

Hardy, J.D., Wolf, H.G., & Goodell, H. (1952). *Pain sensations and reactions.* New York: Hafner Publishing.

Harrison, R.H. (1975). Psychological testing in headache: A review. *Headache, 13,* 177–185.

Hartland, J. (1971). *Medical and dental hypnosis.* London: Bailliere Tindall.

Hendler, N. (1981). *Diagnosis and nonsurgical management of chronic pain.* New York: Raven Press.

Hilgard, E.R. (1980). Hypnosis in the treatment of pain. In Burrows, G.D., & Dennerstein, L. (Eds.), *Handbook of hypnosis and psychosomatic medicine.* Amsterdam: Elsevier/North Holland, pp. 233–267.

Hilgard, E.R., & Hilgard, J.R. (1975). *Hypnosis in the relief of pain.* Los Altos, CA: William Kaufmann.

Holroyd, J., Nuechterlein, K., Shapiro, D., & Ward, F. (1979). Biofeedback and hypnotizability. In Burrows, G.D., Collison, D.R., & Dennerstein, L., *Hypnosis 1979.* Amsterdam: Elsevier/North Holland, pp. 119–131.

Horne, D.J. & Powlett, V. (1980). Hypnotizability and rating scales. In Burrows, G.D., & Dennerstein, L. (Eds.), *Handbook of hypnosis and psychosomatic medicine.* Amsterdam: Elsevier/North Holland, 119–131.

Hunt, S.P., Kelly, J.S., and Emson, P.C. (1980). The electron microscope localization of methionine enkephalin within the superficial layers of the spinal cord. *Neuroscience, 5,* 1871–1890.

International Association for the Study of Pain, Subcommittee on Taxonomy (1979). (H. Merskey, Chair). Pain terms: A list with definitions and notes on usage. *Pain, 6,* 249–252.

Jacobson, E. (1938). *Progressive relaxation.* Chicago: University of Chicago Press.

Jacox, A.K. (1977). Sociocultural and psychological aspects of pain. In Jacox, S. (Ed.), *Pain: A source book for nurses and other health professionals.* Boston: Little Brown, pp. 57–87.

Johnson, M. (1977). Assessment of clinical pain. In Jacox, A. (Ed.), *Pain: A source book for nurses and other health professionals.* Boston: Little Brown, 139–166.

Johnson, R., & Baldwin, D.D., Jr. (1968). Relationship of maternal anxiety to the behavior of young children undergoing dental extraction. *Journal of Dental Research, 47,* 801–805.

Karlin, R., & Morgan, D. (1979). High and moderate hypnotizables: A study of brain function differences in a plateaued sample exposed to colder pressor pain. In Burrows, G.D., Collison, D.R., & Dennerstein, L. (Eds.), *Hypnosis 1979.* Amsterdam: Elsevier/North Holland, pp. 17–24.

Keele, K.D. (1957). *Anatomies of pain.* Springfield, IL: Charles C. Thomas.

Kroger, W.S., & Fezler, W.D. (1976). *Hypnosis and behavior modification: imagery conditioning.* Philadelphia: J.B. Lippincott.

Lazarus, A.A. (1973). Hypnosis as a facilitator in behavior therapy. *International Journal of Clinical and Experimental Hypnosis, 31,* 25–31.

Leavitt, F. (1982). Comparison of three measures for detecting psychological disturbance in patients with low back pain. *Pain, 11,* 299–305.

Lewit, K. (1979). The needle effect in the relief of myofascial pain. *Pain, 6,* 83–90.

Lindblom, U., & Tegner, R. (1979). Are the endorphins active in clinical pain states? Narcotic antagonism in chronic patients. *Pain, 7,* 65–68.

McCaffery, M. (1972). *Nursing management of the patient with pain.* Philadelphia: J.B. Lippincott.

McCaffery, M. (1980). Relieving pain with noninvasive techniques, *Nursing 80, 10,* 55–57.

McCaffery, M. (1981). When your patient's still in pain don't just do something: Sit there. *Nursing 11,* June, 58–61.

McGuire, L. (1981). A short, simple tool for assessing your patient's pain. *Nursing 11,* March, 48–49.

Melzack, R. (1975). The McGill pain questionnaire major properties and scoring methods. *Pain, 1,* 277–299.

Melzack, R., & Wall, P.D. (1965). Pain mechanisms: A new theory. *Science, 150,* 971–979.

Melzack, R., & Wall, P.D. (1982). *The challenge of pain.* New York: Basic Books.

Merskey, H. (1972). Personality traits of patients with chronic pain. *Journal of Psychosomatic Research, 16,* 167–172.

Merskey, H. (1978). Pain and personality. In Sternbach, R.A. (Ed.), *The psychology of pain.* New York: Raven Press, 111–264.

Merskey, H., & Spear, F.G. (1967). *Pain: Psychological and psychiatric aspects.* London: Bailliere, Tindall & Cassel.

Neal, H. (1978). *The politics of pain.* New York: McGraw-Hill.

Needham, F., & Outterson-Wood, T. (1955). Medical use of hypnotism. *British Medical Journal Supplement,* Appendix 10, *190*(1).

Orne, M.T. (1980). On the construct of hypnosis: How its definition affects research and its clinical application. In Burrows, G.D., & Dennerstein, L. (Eds.), *Handbook of hypnosis and psychosomatic medicine.* Amsterdam: Elsevier/North-Holland, pp. 29–51.

Pain: Report of the panel on pain to the National Advisory Neurological and Communicative Disorders and Stroke Council (#79-1979). US Department of Health Education & Welfare, National Institutes of Health, 1979.

Pelletier, K.R. (1977). *Mind as healer, mind as slayer.* New York: Delta.

Pettit, G.A. (1979). Adjunctive trance and family therapy for terminal cancer. In Burrows, G.D., Collison, D.R., & Dennerstein, L. (Eds.), *Hypnosis 1979.* Amsterdam: Elsevier/North Holland, pp. 63–69.

Pilowsky, I. (1978). Psychodynamics of the pain experience. In Sternbach, R.A. (Ed.), *The psychology of pain.* New York: Raven Press, pp. 203–217.

Pilowsky, I., & Spence, N.D. (1976). Illness behavior symptoms associated with intractable pain. *Pain, 2,* 61–71.

Rodger, B.P. (1972). Therapeutic conversation and posthypnotic suggestion. *American Journal of Nursing, 72*(4), 714–717.

Sacerdote, P. (1970). Theory and practice of pain control in malignancy and other protracted or recurring painful illnesses. *International Journal of Clinical and Experimental Hypnosis, 18,* 160–180.

Sacerdote, P. (1980). Hypnosis and terminal illness. In Burrows, G.D. & Dennerstein, L. (Eds.), *Handbook of hypnosis and psychosomatic medicine*. Amsterdam: Elsevier/North Holland, pp. 421–442.

Sarbin, T.R., & Slagle, R. (1980). Psychophysiological outcomes of hypnosis. In Burrows, G.D., and Dennerstein, L. (Eds.), *Handbook of hypnosis and psychosomatic medicine*. Amsterdam: Elsevier/North Holland, 53–65.

Schafer, D.W. (1975). Hypnosis in a burn unit. *International Journal of Clincal and Experimental Hypnosis, 23*, 1–14.

Schluderman, E., & Zubeck, J.P. (1962). Effect of age on pain sensitivity. *Perceptual Motor Skills, 14*, 295.

Shor, R.E. (1972). The fundamental problem in hypnosis research as viewed from historic perspectives. In Fromm, E. & Shor, R.E. (Eds.), *Hypnosis: Research developments and perspectives*. New York: Aldine-Atherton, 15–41.

Snyder, S. (1980). Brain peptides as neurotransmitters. *Science, 209*, 976–983.

Spear, F.G. (1967). Pain in psychiatric patients. *Journal of Psychosomatic Research, 11*, 187–193.

Staub, R., Tursky, B., & Schwartz, G. (1971). Self-control and predictability: Their effects on reactions to aversive stimulation. *Journal of Personality and Social Psychology, 18*(2), 157–162.

Sternbach, R.A. (1968). *Pain: A psychophysiological analysis*. New York: Academic Press.

Sternbach, R.A. (1974). *Pain patients: Traits and treatment*. New York: Academic Press.

Sternbach, R.A. (1978). Clinical aspects of pain. In Sternbach, R.A. (Ed.), *The psychology of pain*. New York: Raven Press.

Stewart, M.L. (1977). Measurement of clinical pain. In Jacox, A.K. (Ed.), *Pain: A source book for nurses and other health professionals*. Boston: Little, Brown, pp. 170–234.

Szasz, T.S. (1957). *Pain and pleasure: A study of bodily feelings*. New York: Basic Books.

Szasz, T.S. (1974). A psychiatric perspective on pain and its control. In Hart, F.D. (Ed.), *The treatment of chronic pain*. England: Medical and Technical Publishing.

Terenius, L. (1979). Endorphins in chronic pain. In Bonica, J.B., Liebeskind, J.R., & Albe-Fessard, D.G. (Eds.), *Advances in pain research and therapy*. New York: Raven Press, 3, 459–471.

Twycross, R.G. (1978). Relief of pain. In Saunders, C.M. (Ed.), *The measurement of terminal disease*. London: Edward Arnold, pp. 65–92.

Wadden, T.A., & Anderton, C.H. (1982). The clinical use of hypnosis. *Psychological Bulletin, 91*(2), 215–243.

Weisenberg, M. (1977a). Cultural and racial reactions to pain. In Weisenberg, M. (Ed.), *The control of pain*. New York: Psychological Dimensions.

Weisenberg, M. (1977b). Pain and pain control. *Psychological Bulletin, 84*(5), 1008–1044.

Weitzenhoffer, A.M. (1972). Behavior therapeutic techniques and hypnotherapeutic models. *American Journal of Clinical Hypnosis, 15*, 71–82.

West, D.A. (1981). Understanding endorphins: Our natural pain relief system. *Nursing, 2*(2), 50.

Wolff, B.B., & Langley, S. (1968). Cultural factors and the response to pain: A review. *American Anthropologist, 70*, 150.

Woodrow, K.M., Friedman, G.G., Siegelaub, A.B., & Collen, M.F. (1972). Pain tolerance: Differences according to age, sex,and race. *Psychosomatic Medicine, 34,* 548.

Zahourek, R.P. (1982a). Hypnosis in nursing practice; emphasis on the 'problem patient' who has pain (part I). *JPNMHS, 20*(3), 13–17.

Zahourek, R.P. (1982b). Hypnosis in nursing practice. Emphasis on the 'problem patient' who has pain (part II). *JPNMHS, 20*(4), 21–24.

Zbrowski, M. (1969). *People in pain.* San Francisco: Jossey-Bass.

Zola, I.K. (1966). Cultures and symptoms—An analysis of patients presenting complaints. *American Sociological Review, 31,* 615–630.

7

Treating Pain with Hypnosis: Two Case Studies

Marcia G. Fishman

When using hypnosis, relaxation or imagery techniques for handling pain, it is usual to assess the patients and their perception of pain first. Realistically, there are times when the process must be greatly abbreviated but even under such circumstances it is often possible to obtain useful information. The following case examples demonstrate how approaches will differ depending on the situation.

Involvement with the first client who had acute pain was a situation in which I as the therapist, managed to meet certain criteria even with the existing urgency. These criteria included (1) establishing rapport and confidence with the patient and her family, (2) making the environment as comfortable as possible, and (3) using information obtained from the patient.

CASE STUDY; ACUTE PAIN CRISIS

I was introduced to Rose and her son through her nurse, who was both a colleague and client of mine, for help with headaches. Rose, a woman in her mid-sixties, had been a strong, independent, and vital person who now was ravaged by her struggle with metastatic thyroid cancer. Even so, I could see there was enough fight left in her to want to try and overcome the intractable pain she now suffered.

We only spent five or ten minutes together, in which Rose and her son asked me how I used "imagery and relaxation" to help her nurse get control of her migraine headaches. I explained that these techniques seem to change the body's physical response to painful stimulation as well as to change one's tolerance to the pain, though the reason was not fully understood. Rose said she needed help, as "Dilaudid every two to three hours was no longer very effective." Rose asked me if I would mind her mentioning these techniques to her physician. I encouraged her to ask him if he would let me be of assistance.

From Rose's son I learned she was now totally bedridden due to severe weakness, multiple pathological fractures (including the pelvis and several ribs), and, of course, the depressing and debilitating pain. Rose realized she did not have much longer to live. However, she did not want to suffer so terribly. This was as much for her son's, daughter-in-law's, and grandchildren's peace of mind, as for her own comfort and dignity.

The next day Rose asked to see me. She seemed visibly embarrassed as she informed me her physician did not think my techniques would be the most effective way to deal with "the pain." She informed me a cordotomy was to be performed the next morning.

Rose was scheduled to be the first surgery in the morning. The physician had written an order that no pain medication be given for six hours before surgery. Rose, her family, and the staff were told it would be the only way to fully evaluate the extent of her pain. Rose felt certain she could endure the discomfort for that period of time, especially knowing that her pain might be ended permanently!

I learned from the primary nurse that the patient and her family had been told that the procedure was not always effective but that Rose was felt to be an excellent candidate for the surgical procedure. They were also informed of the possible side effects which occurred in a small number of patients: paralysis (total or partial) and loss of bladder and/or bowel control). The nurse stressed that Rose and her son were disappointed that she could not try "imagery and relaxation."

Upon hearing this, I approached Rose's physician and asked if he would let me try and see if imagery and relaxation would have any effect on Rose's pain. If it helped, it might prevent or at least put off using such an invasive procedure for pain control. The physician was adamant. He felt such interventions would be ineffective and a waste of time.

When I arrived on the unit the following morning the head nurse told me Rose's surgery had been delayed because of an emergency operation her surgeon was performing. It was now eight hours since Rose had had her last pain medication. Though she was experiencing a great deal of pain, she felt she could tolerate it a while longer.

I became involved with my work until noon time. Then a nursing student urgently informed me the head nurse needed me in Rose's room immediately. Outside her closed door I heard the muffled moans. Her son and daughter-in-law met me, crying, "She can't take it any more. The doctors just saw her and said it would only be a little longer so she should hold on. She can't. Please, try and help."

I was literally pulled into the room. The door locked behind me. Inside, the head nurse and Rose's nurse were trying to comfort her. Her head was twisting from side to side. Rose herself had put a washcloth between her teeth to try and muffle her cries. The nurse was trying to wash the perspiration away. Yet physical and verbal comforts were now in vain.

Rose's pain was so intense she had actually bent the side rails she'd been desperately clutching. Using a firm but gentle tone, I spoke. "Rose, it's Marci, do you remember me?" She shook her head yes. "Good, now listen. I can help you, but you must help me." (She opened her eyes and stopped thrashing about). "That's better." (I now removed the cloth from between her teeth.)

Marci: Rose, think carefully; where is the worst pain?

Rose: In my back, hips, and thighs.

Marci: What does it feel like?

Rose: Crushing, like a huge rope is knotted around these parts being pulled tighter and tighter.

Marci: What would make it feel better?

Rose: Something warm and soothing.

Marci: One more question. Can you describe a favorite place you would like to be right now?

Rose: Are you sure this can help?

Marci: Yes, very sure. Tell me about your favorite place.

Rose: I would be in my favorite chair in my living room looking at the mural of the English rose garden my son painted for me.

Marci: Can I do anything to make you more comfortable in this bed?

Rose: Can I have another pillow under my head?

Marci: Of course. (The other nurses swiftly placed the pillow.) While this was being done, I motioned for her family to be seated nearby. I also dimmed the lights.

Marci: Now Rose, this will be very pleasant and help you feel much more comfortable. Now close your eyes. Imagine yourself sitting comfortably in your favorite chair. Feel the warmth of the rising sun coming through the window penetrating your body. Breathe in and out slowly. In, out, in and out. That's right, nice and easy. There you are sitting quietly and comfortably in your chair. (She released a side rail.) You're doing fine. Let yourself begin to relax.

Rose: I can't, it still hurts too much.

Marci: Can you still imagine yourself sitting in the chair and feel the warmth of the sun?

Rose: Yes.

Marci: Good. And you are beginning to relax. You've released the side rail on your right. Now, let go of the other. Hold my hand instead.

Rose: I may hurt you.

Marci: I promise you won't and it will help us both feel more comfortable. Continue to breathe in and out, nice and easy, calmly. You're doing wonderfully. Rose, I want you to imagine that beautiful mural. Can you see it before you?

Rose: (She nodded yes.)

Marci: Tell me about your very favorite spot in the garden.

Rose: It's the rose bushes in the lower right corner. All shades, reds, yellows, peach. They make me feel good.

Marci: Are you feeling better?

Rose: Yes, but the pain is still so strong.

Marci: But you are stronger! Rose, imagine yourself as a beautiful rose with its petals and leaves very tightly closed in the cool of the early dawn (Her face mirrored the description.) Is that how your back, hips, and legs feel? So tight the pain is unable to escape?

Rose: Oh, yes!

Marci: Rose, you have shown excellent control in describing your pain and discomfort. Now, I'm sure you will have the control to decrease it. Feel the warmth of the rising sun all about you. It's a new day, fresh with energy. Let it penetrate you, slowly warming you. As the healing warmth penetrates the rose, slowly the petals and leaves begin to unfold and relax. Let the warmth of the sun help to open up your petals. That's it, as the petals open you begin to relax. The more you relax and the petals open, the more the pain and discomfort can escape. As the pain subsides, the more relaxed and comfortable you become.

Continue to imagine the soothing warmth of the sun, allowing all of your petals to unfold. When all of the petals are open you will be much more comfortable and able to await your surgery. Keep feeling the sun and letting your petals open. When all of your petals are open, let me know.

(Over the next two minutes, we quietly watched Rose relax. It was visible in her entire facial and body language. She continued to hold my hand but relaxed her grip.)

Rose: All my petals are open and taking in the warmth of the sun.

Marci: How do you feel?

Rose: I still have discomfort, but I can certainly tolerate it.

Marci: Rose, you will be able to tolerate this just by imagining the rose and the healing sun. It will be your control over any terrible pain. When it comes time for the surgery, imagine the setting sun and the petals closing for the night. The pain will increase so the physicians can correctly evaluate you, but the discomfort will not get out of control again. Continue to rest in the sun for now. When you open your eyes, bring the comfort with you. I will count to three. When I get to three, you will open your eyes. One, two, three. Rose opened her eyes. Her son asked how she felt.

Rose: I can stand this discomfort. 'I feel much looser.' Is it alright for me to sleep? I wasn't able to last night.

I assured her she could sleep. If at any time she felt an increase in discomfort, all she had to do was recall the images and sensations she had just experienced.

It was truly amazing that even under such duress Rose was able to concentrate and gain control over her pain. Even at our most vulnerable, we are often far stronger than we feel.

Rose's surgery was successful, and the only untoward effect was constant tingling in her feet, which she gladly tolerated.

Her son told the physician about the episode of imagery and its effect. "Wouldn't it have been worth the try, rather than put my mother through such a horrible period of time, not to mention the greater risk of surgery itself?" The physician still did not feel comfortable with such techniques. "Her decrease in pain during that time could only be attributed to the fact that it was mind over matter."

How did I know it would work? I really didn't. However, I admit when I met Rose an inner strength came through and I felt a positive rapport with her from the start. During the crisis this feeling gave me the confidence and ability to use whatever I had at hand.

I do not negate the effectiveness of cordotomies. However, I strongly prefer to use the least traumatic and invasive technique whenever possible.

I am glad Rose was able to live out her last weeks in relative comfort and dignity, no matter what means it took.

CASE EXAMPLE: CHRONIC PAIN

Pat was a nurse with severe degenerative disc disease (L5-S1) that caused constant and debilitating pain. Along with low back pain she experienced constant radiating pain down the right leg. At times the leg had severe paresthesias and weakness. Though she had returned to work fulltime, only a fair amount of medication made it possible. Cyclobenzaprine (Flexeril), oxycodone (Percodan), and aspirin had all been prescribed to make it possible for her to continue her lifestyle.

I became acquainted with her about one year after her initial diagnosis. Though the pain was much less than during the acute phase, Pat continued to be uncomfortable. The pain was constant, fatiguing, and depressing. Worst of all, she hated the feeling of "always being drugged."

We spent over an hour discussing various methods of pain control and how she felt her pain had interfered with her life. Beside all of the disadvantages mentioned previously was the overwhelming loss of control she experienced. Her physician, physical therapist, medications, pain, and fatigue now regulated her existence.

Pat was able to give me an extensive description of her pain, including location, type, what it would look like, what color it was, even what it would sound like. She also described situations that made it worse, as well as those that lessened the discomfort. Interestingly, Pat definitely saw her pain as orange-red to bright yellow, and very hot, like lightning or an electrical shock. Still, one of the things she felt eased the pain (muscle and nerve spasms) was heat, such as the hot yellow sun. Pat's ideal places for relaxation were beaches and deep forests. During the evaluation period I learned she did not know how to swim and had a fear of being in the water.

My intention was not to have Pat come to me whenever she needed help to control her pain. It was vital to teach her the techniques of relaxation and imagery so she could regain and maintain control over her own life.

From our interview I found Pat to be highly motivated. After the evaluation I reviewed how I would achieve an altered state of consciousness. We then got into the actual practice session. Pat chose to sit in a comfortable chair. I began induction by having her close her eyes, breathing in and out slowly. I set the pace and tone. "In (2, 3, 4) out (2, 3, 4); in (2, 3, 4) out (2, 3, 4), calm (2, 3, 4), quiet (2, 3, 4). As you exhale feel your muscles relax." At this point I asked Pat to concentrate on relaxing specific groups of muscles in a systematic progression throughout her body. It was at this point I could see her relax her right leg from its usual tight, guarded position. She admitted feeling very relaxed and aware of her body. I then asked her to visualize herself lying on her favorite beach with the warm sun on her back. The suggestions were not only focused on decreasing the pain but giving her strength, energy, and an overall sense of well-being. Emphasis was also placed on her having the ability to again take control of her life.

Pat saw me frequently in the beginning. She did not seem to get as much relief when she practiced self hypnosis as when I gave the suggestions. I, however, insisted she continue to practice several times a day on her own, and gradually it became easier for her. It made her much more aware of her body and its responses to daily stress. She began using self hypnosis to decrease the everyday stress, thereby decreasing muscle tension and spasm.

She also found she needed less medication, as the effect seemed to last longer when used in combination with self hypnosis. She also realized because the muscle tension was less she needed a lower dosage of medication. The less drugged she felt, the more energy she had. Within a few weeks she had stopped taking all prescription drugs. She now took these medications only when she overstrained her back, which she tried hard to avoid. She began having an overall feeling of increased well-being. This, in turn, led to more activity and energy. The ability to resume her lifestyle in a more healthy and realistic way gave her back the sense of self-control she needed. There is no denying Pat had to compromise in some areas. She needed to physically rest more, but that she could handle.

I did make a tape for Pat. There are still times she has an exacerbation and seems to respond better to the external suggestion rather than her own inner voice.

It has been 2½ years since Pat first came to me. She now takes only Motrin when her back flares up. She also sees a physical therapist regularly, who has her on an exercise regime. Before, the pain and fatigue were so constant she was not able to maintain any physical exercise routine consistently.

Pat has incorporated self-hypnosis into many phases of her life. Pain control, decreasing daily stress, helping to control tension headaches, and increased energy. Pat is far happier having control over what she is able to realistically achieve. She did not like the physicians telling her, "Do this." "You can't do that." "You must take this medicine." She was especially upset by the fact that physicians were so ready to give her narcotics and tranquilizers for the rest of her life.

SUMMARY

Pain control techniques can be utilized with both acute and chronic situations, and, depending on the patient and his or her problems, can be more or less simplistic. When relief occurs as it did in these cases the satisfaction for both care-giver and patient is marked. These techniques can be effective with or without other means of medical, surgical, or nursing interventions.

—————————— 8 ——————————

Hypnosis and Anesthesia

Louis R. McCoy

Anesthesia is a combination of art and science; so is hypnosis. Hypnosis has been a part of medicine throughout the centuries, and it was found to be an effective method of inducing anesthesia long before the existence of chemical anesthesia. The mind, stimulated by suggestion, is capable of great things. As a result of various emotional reactions, remarkable physical and mental changes can occur; these same changes can be obtained through hypnosis. (McCoy 1974)

HISTORICAL BACKGROUND

Hypnosis has been used by virtually every culture and race of people. In Biblical times, people went to "sleep temples" to be cured of their illnesses by the Egyptian priests. The ancient Chinese employed hypnotic techniques in the form of prayer and meditation. There is evidence that "magic sleep" was used for various purposes by the Romans. The Greeks unknowingly used hypnosis, thinking that cures came from the gods. Hippocrates wrote about impressing health on the ill by inducing trances and making passes over the body. (Udolf 1981)

Throughout the centuries, many great medical men have studied, researched, and experimented with hypnosis. They usually were labeled charlatans, quacks, or impostors. Hypnosis gained a great deal of popularity and acceptance during World Wars I and II and the Korean conflict when the need arose to rapidly treat war neuroses. On September 13, 1958, after much research, the American Medical Association officially accepted hypnosis as a "tool" to be used by the medical profession. The association strongly recommended that instruction in the use of hypnosis be included in the curricula of medical schools. (Kroger 1977)

CLINICAL APPLICATION OF HYPNOSIS

By the last decades of the nineteenth century, there was no longer any question as to the reality of hypnosis, and its use in producing analgesia and anesthesia was no longer an experiment. Historically, natural or hypnoanesthesia preceded chemical anesthesia by approximately 21 years.

The first operation using hypnoanesthesia reported in the United States was a nasal polypectomy, performed 13 years before Crawford Long started using ether as an anesthetic agent. To date, virtually every body cavity has been entered and almost every organ has been operated on using hypnoanesthesia. Review of the medical literature since 1970 reveals numerous valid reports of surgical procedures performed under hypnoanesthesia.

In order to use hypnosis for anesthesia more effectively, it is important to understand that hypnosis is a method or technique, not an anesthetic agent. Hypnosis will never replace chemical anesthesia, because not all patients can be hypnotized as easily as they can be anesthetized. Nevertheless, hypnosis can be very useful before, during, and after the surgical procedure.

There are two ways hypnosis can be used in an anesthesia practice. First, hypnosis may be used by itself without any chemical agents of any kind. This is called *formal hypnosis* or *hypnoanesthesia*. This method usually requires several sessions with the patient prior to the scheduled procedure. During the hypnotic sessions, the patient is prepared for the anticipated procedure, both psychologically and physiologically. The patient is conditioned with hypnotic suggestions to produce anesthesia (numbness) in the area where the procedure is to be performed. The age progression technique (APT) is used to take the patient through the entire procedure mentally while in the hypnotic state. Once the patient has visualized the event mentally, he or she then has a memory of everything being normal and the procedure being completed successfully.

In contrast to chemical anesthesia, hypnoanesthesia or formal hypnosis has the advantage of being completely safe and harmless to the patient. The disadvantage of using this method is time. In order to use hypnosis as the sole and total means of producing anesthesia, or even as the major portion of the anesthetic procedure, more time generally is required than just the preanesthetic visit the night before surgery. Though it may very well be the anesthesia method of choice for many patients, it is not used frequently for two reasons: (1) it is estimated that less than 1 percent of the population could undergo a major surgical procedure using just hypnosis, and (2) anesthesia personnel often do not have the time required for conditioning the patient properly prior to the proposed procedure. The basic induction of hypnosis alone can require as long as 10 to 15 minutes.

The second way to use hypnosis in an anesthesia practice is called *narcohypnosis*. This is the most commonly used method in an anesthesia practice today. This method combines the use of hypnotic techniques with chemical anesthesia agents. The advantage of using this combination, is to reduce the amount of chemical agents used. Experience has demonstrated that the amount of chemical agents required can be reduced by 75 to 85 percent. By using less of the chemical agents, depression of the cardiovascular, pulmonary, renal and hepatic systems is greatly reduced. Because of this fact, the patient benefits from a smooth and safe anesthesia, and the recovery period is much shorter. At least one hypnotic session is required preoperatively, at which time the APT is accomplished. The patient is then hypnotized again immediately prior to the chemical anesthetic induction (Guerra & Aldrette 1980).

How does the anesthetist actually decide when to use hypnoanesthesia or narcohypnosis? The decision is generally resolved by the attitude of the patient and the attending physician. All available information regarding the patient's mental and physical condition and the planned procedure must be carefully evaluated. The final determination is made exactly as it would be if chemical anesthesia were to be used without hypnosis.

From all this, it would appear that hypnosis is an ideal method of anesthesia for most operations. Why is it not used more widely? The answer is that although the technical aspects of inducing hypnosis are easy to learn, successful induction and maintenance of hypnoanesthesia depends largely upon the interaction of many factors in the personalities of the patient and hypnotherapist. In addition to this, the number of anesthesia personnel properly trained and qualified to use hypnosis in their anesthesia practice is limited.

In addition to the benefits previously mentioned for anesthesia, there are many other benefits to be derived from the use of hypnotic suggestions:

1. Helping the patient to overcome fear, apprehension, and anxiety associated with the anticipated anesthesia and surgery, thereby increasing patient cooperation.
2. Sedation, either in conjunction with or as a substitute for drug medication.
3. Increased patient cooperation and create peace of mind.
4. A more pleasant and comfortable postoperative period, including (a) reduced incidence of postoperative nausea and vomiting, (b) better deep breathing and necessary coughing, (c) a raised pain threshold, which reduces the need for narcotics, (d) earlier fluid intake, and (e) increased urinary output.
5. Fewer postoperative complications and faster recovery.
6. Producing amnesia of the procedure.

7.   Establishing better morale, thus motivating the patient toward a faster recovery. (Hilgard, Hilgard 1975)

HYPNOSIS FOR HOSPITALIZED PATIENTS

The hospitalized patient is generally an excellent candidate for hypnosis. Simply by being admitted to the hospital, the patient is already in a slightly altered state of consciousness, by having focused attention to the inner feelings that are aroused by being in a strange environment. A person in this state is motivated to participate in the hypnotic process. The patient who is so motivated will pay attention to anything the anesthetist might suggest to increase comfort and decrease stress and tension.

Hypnosis can be used as the method of anesthesia for any surgical, obstetrical, or dental procedure on a patient of almost any age. It is useful in emergency rooms for minor surgical and orthopedic procedures, especially when the patient has just eaten a heavy meal. When utilizing hypnosis for major procedures, it has proved to be more beneficial when used as an adjunct to chemical agents.

HYPNOSIS FOR OUTPATIENT SURGERY

Performing surgery on an outpatient basis in an office or clinic environment is becoming very common in certain areas of the country. This has been necessitated mainly by the increase in hospital costs. Outpatient surgery can be safely performed in a properly equipped and staffed outpatient facility at a considerable financial saving for the patient. An office or clinic surgical unit is an ideal place to use hypnosis in conjunction with conventional anesthesia.

Prior to the date of the scheduled outpatient surgery, the patient meets with the anesthetist/hypnotherapist. During this visit, the procedure to be followed on the day of surgery is explained in detail, and all questions the patient has regarding the procedure are answered. The patient is then hypnotized (relaxed), and is taken "mentally" through the entire surgical procedure by the use of direct suggestions and visual imagery techniques. This session usually requires approximately 30 to 45 minutes. The patient enjoys the relaxation and feels much less tense and anxious about the proposed surgery. The patient is instructed to repeat the relaxation technique at home each night until the day of surgery.

When the patient arrives at the outpatient facility on the day of the surgery, the anesthetist/hypnotherapist hypnotizes (relaxes) the patient again and reinforces the suggestions given previously. As a result of the hypnotic suggestions, the patient is more relaxed and less apprehensive, thus requiring much less chemical anesthesia. Depending on the motivation of the patient, hypnosis may be used as the sole method of anesthesia. (McCoy 1974)

CONCLUSION

Hypnosis is a valuable addition to the methods and techniques available to the anesthetist. It is a safe and uncomplicated method of anesthesia, to be used only by competent, skillful, and ethical anesthetists within the limitations of their specialty and in the best interests of their patients. Ideal anesthesia can be achieved by combining hypnotic techniques with less chemical agents, for the same results with fewer risks to the patient. Instruction in the use of hypnosis should be included in all medical and anesthesia educational programs. As more people become educated in the subject, it will become more readily and widely accepted and used.

REFERENCES

Guerra, F., & Aldrette, J.A. (1980). *Emotional and psychological responses to anesthesia and surgery.* New York: Grune & Stratton.

Hilgard, E., & Hilgard, J.R. (1975). *Hypnosis in the relief of pain.* Los Altos, CA: William Kaufman.

Kroger, W.S. (1977). *Clinical and experimental hypnosis* (ed. 2), Philadelphia: J.B. Lippincott.

McCoy, L.R. (1974). Hypnosis—its relationship to anesthesia. *AANA Journal, 42;* 227–232.

Udolf, R. (1981). *Handbook of hypnosis for professionals.* New York: Van Nostrand-Reinhold.

PART III

Clinical Applications: Working with Women and Children

9

Hypnosis in Obstetrics and Gynecology

Barbara J. Smith

Mythologically, women are supposed to suffer during pregnancy, labor, and delivery. Gynecological problems and genital examinations have also been viewed as women's private "curse." While the mythology still holds, particularly in some socioeconomic and cultural groups, the western medical profession is seeking to change these ideas. We now encourage women to have preventive examinations, obtain early treatment for disorders, and to have safe, prepared, and comfortable childbirth. Hypnosis has been found to be a safe and rewarding tool to help women be as comfortable as possible during pregnancy, labor, and delivery. Patients who are anxious, who refuse pain medication or anesthesia, or who are phobic or experiencing panic related to gynecological examinations are also good candidates for the use of hypnotic techniques.

This chapter explores the use of hypnotic techniques with gynecological and obstetrical patients. The primary techniques and theoretical frameworks are explained, followed by case examples with a problematic obstetrical patient, an antenatal group, two cases of hyperemesis gravidarium, and a patient fearful of inserting a vaginal applicator. Kroger's method, which is primarily used, and the process, problems, and issues are explored. While the case examples focus on pathological situations, these techniques are also useful in normal obstetrical and gynecological situations.

THEORETICAL FRAMEWORK

Kroger (1963) hypothesized that appropriate hypnotherapy can relieve anxiety responsible for many psychogenic symptoms by altering faulty attitudes of femininity and sexuality. Furthermore, hypnoanesthesia can alleviate many psychosomatic conditions in obstetrics, such as dyspyrunia, and of course, is appropriate for use in normal labor and delivery. Kroger advocated hypnosis with other methods to obtain best results; e.g., hypnoanesthesia combined with chemoanesthesia can substantially lessen the pain of parturition. Hypnosis relieves the psychogenic component responsible for nausea and vomiting in early pregnancy. Hypnosis and/or strong suggestions are valuable in the prevention of habitual abortion; miscarriage can be prevented in properly selected patients if placental separation has not occurred, by diminishing the strength and the frequency of the uterine contractions. Kroger claimed hypnosis effectively treats heartburn, promotes lactation, and curbs the "eating for two" syndrome often responsible for weight gain and subsequent preeclampsia and toxemia. Additionally, hypnosis produces relaxation in highly anxious patients undergoing pelvic examinations. (Kroger, 1963).

HYPNOSIS IN OBSTETRICS

Comparison of Hypnosis and Lamaze in Childbirth

Tension and fear cause muscle tension and intensified pain during labor and delivery. Both distraction and relaxation interrupt the pain–tension–pain cycle. In addition to relaxation, both hypnosis and the Lamaze childbirth method serve to raise the patient's pain threshold through learning and suggestion (Kroger, 1963). The Lamaze method is a physical and psychological preparation for childbirth based on conditioning, concentration, discipline, and education about the birth process. Through prescribed exercises, practice, and coaching the woman becomes educated, less fearful, and conditioned to relaxation and distraction when confronting pain. Controlled specialized breathing augments this process. Due to the stress of labor, the nature of the relaxation and breathing exercises, the suggestions given during classes, and the repetitive nature of the practice, the woman may enter an altered (trance) state spontaneously.

The Lamaze method strongly resembles the hypnotic process. Training in hypnosis, however, may use vivid imagery for distraction, glove anesthesia for pain, specific suggestions, and deepening techniques, none of which are incorporated into Lamaze training. Furthermore, the goal in using hypnosis is an altered state of consciousness, which is not the aim with Lamaze training.

The author has found that the most positive results are obtained when hypnosis is combined with Lamaze breathing exercises. With the Lamaze method the woman is instructed to take a deep breath when a contraction begins. When using hypnosis, the author suggests that with each deep breath she will go deeper and deeper into trance and will feel more comfortable and relaxed.

Training in Hypnosis, Autohypnosis, and Glove Anesthesia

The specific process of hypnotherapy is as follows. Kroger posits that hypnotic conditioning should begin during the third or fourth month of pregnancy. During this period, the patient is trained in autohypnosis and glove anesthesia and is educated about the birth process. At each session, posthypnotic suggestions emphasize that the patient need not have any more discomfort than she is willing to bear. Repeated suggestions, relaxation exercises, and conditioning techniques help the patient reach deeper states of hypnosis over time and raise her pain threshold (Kroger, 1963).

In training for hypnosis and autohypnosis, the patient is seen weekly until her pain threshold is raised to the level that will permit her to have a pleasant experience during labor and delivery. First, a hypnotic response is induced, then this response is speeded up until the patient is able to achieve a medium or deep trance in a few seconds at a given signal. The signal to induce hypnosis instantly is as follows: "Breathe deeply and relax at the count of three, one . . . two . . . three." The nurse suggests when the patient has any discomfort, it will be relieved by the signal of raising her finger.

Next, glove anesthesia for one or both hands is taught while the patient is in a deep hypnotic state. She is told,

> As you touch your hand, it will feel numb, like you feel when you have been sitting on your hand. When you feel this numbness, your hand will be anesthetized, and you can use this hand throughout labor and delivery to relieve pain in a particular area. As you rub this hand over your abdomen or imagine you are touching your perineum with this hand, you will have transferred the numbness from your hand to your abdomen or perineum." Furthermore, the patient is told, "With every breath you take, you will go deeper and deeper into a relaxed state. You can remove your hand and the area you have touched will become numb and anesthetized and the hand will become normal.

Instantaneous anesthesia, in response to signal, is accomplished under hypnosis. Practice and conditioning achieve posthypnotic anesthesia. Finally, an anesthetic response to a signal is established while the patient is in a waking state. The physical act of the patient entering the hospital can be an additional signal for the patient to become relaxed. For a step-by-step explanation of autohypnosis training, see Appendix III at the end of the book.

Case Example: Hypnosis for Antepartum, Labor, Delivery, and Postpartum Period

A 21-year-old white woman was seven months pregnant when she began psychotherapy and hypnotherapy because she had many fears related to the pregnancy. She was uneducated and unsophisticated about her anatomy and the birth process. She feared dying in childbirth, hemorrhaging, dropping her newborn baby, and being unable to void after delivery and having to be catheterized. Nearly phobic of receiving any medication or anesthesia during labor and delivery, she expressed a desire to be alert throughout. She was terrified a doctor would remove parts of her body during childbirth. She assumed the physician had removed her liver after he delivered her first baby. She claimed ignorance that the placenta was delivered normally after the birth of the child. Evidence of these fears occurred when she presented me with several newspaper clippings. "TV Health Warning for Women" and "Life, Death, and the American Woman" emphasized death in childbirth. Another article, "Anesthesia Kills Boy, 13" described how a boy with a fractured elbow died because of a freakish reaction to a common anesthetic. The patient felt both articles were related to her outcome. Discussing how these articles related to her own labor and delivery was vital to the hypnotherapeutic process. Such seemingly unusual and personalized anxieties highlight the importance of utilizing hypnosis within the context of a therapeutic relationship.

The patient had a past positive experience with hypnosis and was willing to learn autohypnosis. She was seen weekly during the last two months of her pregnancy. She also attended natural childbirth classes. During the hypnotic sessions she was given "external images" of the birth process through educational material concerning labor and delivery. She was encouraged to use glove anesthesia in conjunction with autohypnosis and was reassured that the physician was aware of her problems. The physician and therapist maintained a close working relationship with the patient. She was given a tour of the labor room, delivery room, and postpartum ward, and was introduced to the staff. She was comforted knowing that the therapist would remain with her during labor and delivery.

During hypnotherapy sessions, imagery of pleasant experiences, especially a trip the patient had taken to the Caribbean, was used to promote relaxation. At one session, while the patient was in a deep hypnotic trance, the therapist discussed the patient's fear about holding and dropping a small baby using the following hallucinatory experience to rehearse a therapeutic change (Rossi, 1980):

Now listen carefully; I will tell you 12 things you must do, one at a time, without becoming panicky:

1. You must open your eyes slowly and widely.
2. You will see a beautiful baby on the desk.
3. You will stand up.
4. You will walk over to the desk.
5. You will look at the baby.
6. You will smile and play with the baby.
7. You will pick up the baby.
8. You will walk back to your chair and sit down as you hold the baby.
9. You will practice holding and cuddling the baby as a pleasant and relaxing experience.

10. You will say out loud, "I am not afraid to hold a baby; I am relaxed."
11. You will stand up, walk back to the desk with the baby and place it on the desk.
12. You will return to your seat, sit down, close your eyes and remain relaxed. When you are alert, you will remember the positive experience of holding a baby without fear of dropping it and will not experience this fear again.

The patient was given another posthypnotic suggestion that she would recall what she wanted to remember about the experience and then was dehypnotized. Later she stated the experience was good; she saw herself holding the baby, was not afraid, and believed that she would be comfortable holding her baby. She was surprised about the whole experience.

Hypnosis and posthypnotic suggestions were used during the antepartum period to establish that after delivery the patient would (1) feel alert and better than any other patient on the ward; (2) not experience any afterbirth pains; (3) use glove anesthesia and transmit it to any area of major discomfort; (4) void two hours after delivery without difficulty; (5) move her bowels 24 hours after delivery without difficulty; (6) comfortably hold and feed her baby; and (7) walk and sit without any discomfort; (8) be discharged within five days without any postpartum difficulties.

During labor the patient refused to take any injection for pain but accepted a paracervical and transvaginal pudenal block. Hypnosis, breathing exercises, and imagery of past pleasant experiences were used to take the place of active painful contractions. This technique proved to be effective in allaying pain and anxiety. The patient was gratified that she had experienced childbirth under hypnosis and had been alert at the birth.

GROUP TRAINING IN HYPNOSIS

Group training in hypnoanesthesia is time saving (Kroger, 1963). Patients identify and empathize with each other and motivation is enhanced by this and by the spirit of competition. This method can be ideal for the busy obstetrical nurse and utilizes concepts and methods standard to group process and group dynamic theoretical frameworks.

Case Example: Group Hypnosis During the Antepartum Period

A group was formed for training five extremely anxious patients in group hypnosis during the antepartum period. The group members were high-risk, unmarried, primiparas, 14 to 18 years old. Each was six to seven months pregnant at the onset of the group. The group members could identify with each other because their problems were similar. The therapist screened, interviewed, and explained hypnosis to each individually. All were receptive.

At the first group meeting, they appeared very uncomfortable. It was difficult to initiate any discussion about their problems. Araoz (1979) stated, "The first modality involved using hypnosis simultaneously with all group members is to encourage communication, either during or after the trance" (p. 4).

Two meetings were spent becoming acquainted, asking questions and learning about hypnosis and autohypnosis. Rules were set and agreed upon, and phone numbers were shared. Then the patients were encouraged to discuss their problems, be supportive, and offer constructive suggestions to each other. If a patient missed a meeting, one of the group members was encouraged to leave the group temporarily to telephone the member to see if she was all right. The members were urged to communicate with one another by phone as a network system. Each was to alert at least one group member and the therapist when labor began, and that group member would call another member, etc., until the entire group was notified. Visits to the maternity ward after the delivery were also recommended to the group members.

At the third session, hypnosis was introduced, and the birth process was described, as well as what they could expect during their group practice sessions. Anxiety-reduction techniques by imagery conditioning were also described. During induction, improved breath control for relaxation was achieved by using rhythmic and syllable-timed speech. The suggestion, "with each breath you take, the deeper relaxed you will feel," was given during each induction and encouraged this control. Images using breathing and relaxation were effective in training these women to perform proper breathing during labor and delivery. The group hypnosis increased the members' self-image, gave them confidence and strength, assisted them in learning to lessen their anxieties, helped them to form a supportive network during a stressful period, and enabled them to prepare for a pleasant experience—labor and delivery with hypnosis.

Four of the five members used autohypnosis successfully and achieved subsequent comfort during labor and delivery. All felt the experience was positive whether or not chemical anesthesia was used in addition.

HYPNOSIS FOR HYPEREMESIS GRAVIDARIUM

Nausea, vomiting, and even hyperemesis gravidarium are astonishingly susceptible to hypnosis. In predisposed individuals, the gastrointestinal tract is symbolically utilized as a way of showing disgust by vomiting. Many women who experience vomiting during pregnancy have been found to have an aversion toward sex or an overdependent attachment to their mothers, and a history of "rejection dyspepsia."

Treatment should be directed toward the patient as a whole, not just toward the symptom. The judicious use of hypnotherapy to understand the need for the symptom, combined with adequate medical management, is indicated for all cases of hyperemesis gravidarium. This often has obviated the need for therapeutic abortion (Kroger, 1963).

Case Examples

A 27-year-old woman who was three months pregnant had severe anxiety and hyperemesis gravidarium. This was her second pregnancy within a year, and hyperemesis gravidarium had caused the first to be terminated by therapeutic abortion. She stated that she had always had a nervous stomach, but physical examinations and tests were always negative for pathology. She had numerous fears about pregnancy and childbirth, which included never being able to stop vomiting, experiencing labor pain, being alone during labor and delivery, and hemorrhaging to death during delivery. She also feared her husband would leave her because of the vomiting, although he was very supportive to her through this crisis. She would not allow her husband to touch her body or to make any sexual overtures once she found out she was pregnant. She became angry and hostile to him and withdrew from everyone close to her. She cried out for her deceased mother many times. The husband felt helpless and did not know how to help her. The couple agreed to see me in family therapy.

The couple was seen weekly during the patient's ante-partum period to improve their communication patterns and to permit restructuring. In individual therapy sessions with her, hypnosis was used for relaxation. During these sessions, imagery, breathing exercises, and posthypnotic suggestions were introduced, as well as autohypnosis training. A taped recording of training for autohypnosis was made specifically for the patient, using imagery of the birth process and other educational material. She was reassured under hypnosis and on the tape that there was no organic component or physical reason for her vomiting. An ego-enhancing suggestion was incorporated onto the tape recording to increase the patient's self-confidence and strength and thereby help her to stop vomiting.

She played the tape at least three times a day to help her relax and to become familiar with the conditioning and the posthypnotic suggestions. One of the specific posthypnotic suggestions was, "I will not vomit during therapy sessions." The therapist's office was the only place where the patient never vomited (Smith, 1982). The suggestion was later increased to, "I will not vomit any more during this pregnancy." These were the only times that any emphasis was placed on the vomiting. The patient resented this lack of emphasis, and it became an issue. It was made clear to her that the purpose of the family sessions was to deal with the problems at hand, not the vomiting. When the patient finally accepted this (after much resistance), she became more receptive to the hypnosis and the vomiting ceased.

Hypnosis was used throughout the antepartum period, labor, and delivery. The patient's husband and the therapist remained with the patient during labor and worked very closely with the patient's physician in making it a pleasant experience. Even though many individuals were interested in the outcome, those who participated in the birthing process were limited to the essential people—father, hypnotist/nurse and physician. (Vadurro and Butts, 1982, p. 623) The patient experienced an uneventful delivery with the use of hypnoanesthesia, breathing exercises, and a combination of paracervical and transvaginal pudenal block, which are ideal for painless childbirth.

A 26-year-old married primipara was admitted to the hospital for the third time in one month for hyperemesis gravidarium. In her third trimester of pregnancy, she verbalized numerous fears related to the pregnancy and some ambivalent feelings about being pregnant. The patient stated she was experiencing marital difficulties resulting from her overdependency on mother, who hated her husband. The patient's mother spent all of her free time visiting the patient at home or at the hospital. She constantly criticized the patient's husband, who, in her view, neglected his wife who was sick and vomiting. The mother antagonized the husband by calling him at work to complain about his lack of involvement in his wife's pregnancy. As a result, the patient's vomiting increased and the husband withdrew more. The patient's mother blamed the physician's inadequate treatment for her daughter's continued vomiting. The patient felt caught between her mother, her husband, and her doctor. At this point, she asked her physician for a psychiatric evaluation. The physician contacted a therapist to assess the situation and make recommendations.

The patient was seen by the therapist daily during her hospital stay. The patient was certain that her vomiting was psychological and was associated with her lifelong overdependency on her mother. She felt it was difficult to break those bonds and that her mother would never let her live her own life. She claimed that she was desperate and wanted help with the problems. The idea of hypnosis was introduced, as well as the suggestion of a family session involving herself, her physician, her husband, both parents, and the therapist to discuss the issues and set therapeutic goals. The patient was afraid to ask her mother for fear of upsetting her. The physician spoke to the patient's parents and they agreed to the family session, as did the patient's husband. However, during the session there was considerable resistance from all family members, which they were encouraged to verbalize by discussing their anger and feelings about the present situation. This was recommended so that all issues would be in the open and dealt with effectively in a protective setting for the group. Hopefully, the group would be able to solve the problem or to come to a mutual understanding and agreement on dealing with the problem. The goal was set that the meeting would not adjourn until a resolution was achieved, regardless of how long it took. Each group member was encouraged to be honest and to not be concerned if his or her feelings were negative about another member, as these would be dealt with within the therapeutic milieu.

Support and confrontation were used as indicated. The group members felt able to ventilate honestly, and the 2 1/2 hour meeting was intense. The group came to an agreement and the patient's mother announced that they would deal with the problems in the following manner: (1) the patient would strive more toward independence; (2) the mother would give her space to be independent; (3) the parents would express more respect to the patient's husband and accept him into the family unit; and (4) the husband would try to form an accepting relationship with the mother and father and spend more supportive time with his wife. At the end of the session everyone was crying. The enormous tension in the room lifted as the mother got up and reached for her son-in-law, apologizing to him and stating how difficult it had been for her to let go of her daughter. He returned her embrace and cried that he wanted them to be his family too and was sorry for how he had acted. Then he reached for the father and they both exchanged apologies. Finally the husband and patient held each other crying. As the group regained control of themselves, the mother thanked the therapist for bringing them together because they would have never done it on their own. They all agreed that the burden they had placed on the patient was related to her vomiting. They decided if problems arose in the future, they would talk about them. The mother said strongly, "I am going away on a long vacation for the first time now, because I never felt I could leave my daughter alone before now." The group laughed and disbanded.

The patient was given a tape recording on training in autohypnosis to use at home. Three months later she delivered healthy twins. She was seen one other time after her discharge from the hospital, and she appeared more relaxed. She had been using hypnosis, the family tension had lessened, and she had stopped vomiting.

CLINICAL USES OF HYPNOSIS IN GYNECOLOGY

Case Example: Hypnosis During Insertion of Vaginal Applicator

A 23-year-old single, shy, young woman whom I have known for many years, was attending law school when she developed a fungal infection in her vagina. She had gone to two physicians for treatment and panicked each time, refusing a vaginal examination. Neither doctor was able to calm the patient, and therefore neither was able to perform the examination. The second doctor, however, gave the patient a prescription for a vaginal cream that had to be inserted vaginally. After she failed at numerous attempts to insert the medication, she panicked and telephoned me long distance to discuss the problem. Because I had known her for many years, she trusted me and turned to me for help. She gradually calmed down and was able to listen to what I had to say. She was willing to try anything, she said, because she was so uncomfortable. I discussed the trial use of hypnosis to enable her to relax enough to insert the applicator, if she would be able to come visit me for the weekend. She agreed to this plan.

When the patient arrived at my home, I explained hypnosis, glove anesthesia, and autohypnosis, and answered her questions about its use. I gave her a 20-minute tape on autohypnosis and asked her to go into a quiet room alone to listen to the tape several times for conditioning, resting between each playing. When she felt she was relaxed enough to attempt insertion of the applicator, she would call me to enter the room. She was instructed to have the applicator ready with the medication on it. When she was ready, I inducted her into a deep trance and used the following imagery:

> I want you to imagine that you are about to insert the applicator into your vagina. You are very relaxed. Your vaginal muscles are very relaxed. Your hand feels anesthesized and numb; you must take your hand and use glove anesthesia so that you can transfer the feeling from your hand to your vagina. Now, hold up your second finger on your left hand when you feel that the muscle in the vagina feels numb and that you are ready to insert the applicator. Your hand feels normal now. Now, I want you to insert the applicator.

The patient was able to insert the applicator and push the plunger in with the medication. I instructed her to remove the applicator and gave her a posthypnotic suggestion that she would use autohypnosis to relax herself. Dehypnotized, she felt that it had been a positive experience and that she would be able to do it herself in the future.

Case Example: Hypnosis During Pelvic Examination

A 21-year-old woman was referred to the psychiatric liaison consultation service by the physician in the obstetrical clinic. Five months into gestation, she had a pathological fear of pelvic or genital contact. A liaison psychiatrist on the team evaluated her and recommended that hypnosis with supportive psychotherapy be used during pelvic examination, antepartum care, and delivery.

A lengthy prehypnosis discussion was held with the patient to answer questions, dispel myths, and provide explanations. She was willing to try hypnosis and autohypnosis if it would relax her. We agreed on a contract for regular hypnotic sessions to prepare her to relax enough to have a pelvic examination and an enjoyable birth.

The patient had a 2 1/2-year-old son and was currently separated from her husband because of their sexual difficulties. She described her first pregnancy as traumatic, mentioning having been held down by the staff while the physician tried to do a pelvic examination. She had not received any prenatal care and entered the hospital in labor, refusing to be examined. She stated, "My marriage has not been properly consummated." For the present pregnancy, the patient had gone to several doctors before coming to this hospital. She felt rejected that none of these doctors wanted to accept her as a patient when she told them about her fears and anxieties related to childbirth.

Her background included an incident of rape at age 9. She had managed to block out all memories of the event until her mother, a diagnosed manic–depressive, discussed the incident with her three years ago. As a rehearsal for the actual examination, the patient was inducted into a deep trance. The following suggestions were then given to the patient:

> You will now open your legs as wide as you can. After they are open, lift them and place them into the stirrups. You will remain relaxed, and with each breath you take, it will be more easy for you to relax your legs and keep them open. You will go deeper and deeper into a state of relaxation. Now you will open your legs as wide as you can, and take a deep breath as the doctor is preparing to examine you. You are fully relaxed, not afraid, but confident, courageous, and ready to be examined. Listen carefully, when I give the word to you to give permission to the doctor, you will open your eyes, but will not be alert, just relaxed. You will tell the doctor these words, "I am ready to be examined now." Now open your eyes . . . there is the doctor.

The patient was able to have a hallucinatory experience by seeing the doctor and giving her permission for him to examine her. Her accepting the validity of a hallucinatory experience indicated that profound hypnotic depth had been achieved.

It took three trials before an effective actual examination could be completed, because the patient would draw her knees together. Deepening techniques eventually relaxed her. The patient was encouraged under hypnosis to use autohypnosis the next time she had to have an examination of any type to relax herself. The patient was dehypnotized and given the suggestion she would remember the experience positively. She was able to use autohypnosis to relax herself for her next examination.

DISCUSSION

Hypnosis in gynecology and obstetrics is proving to be an effective tool in allaying many women's anxieties and discomforts. Hypnosis enables the patient to relax and thereby have a more pleasant experience. Hypnosis can be used in conjunction with chemoanesthesia, the Lamaze method, or alone for comfortable childbirth and numerous gynecological procedures. The cases presented in this chapter were all of patients with a psychological overlay. However, hypnosis can be equally effective with patients in normal deliveries and undergoing regular gynecological procedures.

REFERENCES

Araoz, D.L. (1979). Hypnosis in group therapy. *International Journal of Clinical and Experimental Hypnosis, 27*(1), 4.

Cheek, D., & LeCron, L. (1968). *Clinical hypnotherapy.* New York: Grune & Stratton.

Davenport-Slack, B. (1975). Obstetrical hypnosis and natural childbirth: A comparative evaluation. *International Journal of Clinical and Experimental Hypnosis, 23,* 266–281.

DeVore, J.S. (1979). Psychological anesthesia for obstetrics. In Schnider & Levinson, G. (Eds.), *Anesthesia for obstetrics.* Baltimore: Williams & Wilkins, pp. 65–73.

Hilgard, E., & Hilgard, J. (1975). *Hypnosis in the relief of pain.* Los Altos, CA: William Kaufman.

Johnson, J.M. (1980). Teaching self-hypnosis in pregnancy, labor and delivery. *Maternal Child Nursing, 5,* 98–101.

Kroger, W.S. (1963). *Clinical and experimental hypnosis.* Philadelphia: J.B. Lippincott.

Kroger, W., & Fezler, W. (1976). *Hypnosis and behavior modification: Imagery conditioning.* Philadelphia: J.B. Lippincott.

Smith, B.J. (1981). Consultant advocate for the medically ill hospitalized patient. *Nursing Forum, 20*(2), 115–122.

Smith, B.J. (1982). Management of the patient with hyperemesis gravidarium in family therapy with hypnotherapy as an adjunct. *Journal of the New York State Nursing Association, 20*(1), 17–26.

Sweeney, S. (1978). Relaxation. In Carlson, C.E., & Blackwell, B. (Eds.) *Behavioral concepts and nursing intervention* (ed. 2). Philadelphia: J.B. Lippincott.

Vadurro, J., & Butts, P. (1982). Reducing the anxiety and pain of childbirth through hypnosis. *American Journal of Nursing, 82*(4), 623.

Zahourek, R.P. (1982). Hypnosis in nursing practice—emphasis on the "problem patient" who has pain (part I). *Journal Psychosocial Nursing and Mental Health Services, 20*(3), 15.

10

Self-Hypnosis and Hypnotherapy with Children

Jeanine L. LaBaw and Wallace L. LaBaw

Despite the fact that hypnosis has been utilized with children at least since the 18th century, many professionals remain unaware of children's responsiveness to hypnotic techniques. This chapter will discuss the factors that affect the hypnotizability of children, the role of the pediatric nurse as the hypnotherapist, specific induction techniques for children, and case examples illustrating the authors' combined 34 years of experience working in the field of hypnosis.

HYPNOTIC RESPONSIVITY IN CHILDREN

Historical Perspective

It is likely that hypnosis was first used with children in primitive cultures, where they were included in rites that incorporated rhythmical music, dancing, hallucinations, and trances. One of the first recorded accounts of the use of hypnosis with children in Western culture occured in the writings of Franz Mesmer (Shor & Orne, 1965) in the 18th century. Mesmer proposed a therapy process involving light touches and passing of the hands various distances from the body. The reasons for Mesmer's success, contact, imagery, and imitation, are some of the same tools which we currently use to induce trance in children. Subsequently, Dr. John Elliotson cited the use of "mesmerism" to extract teeth from children without discomfort. Auguste Liebault and Hippolyte Bernheim investigated hypnosis at the School of Nancy in the late 1800s and found that children were quickly and easily hypnotized. They carried out normative studies, and compiled data from 755 subjects, and discovered that there were no differences in hypnotizability based on sex, and that children ages 7 to 14 seemed to be the most hypnotizable. No children ages 14 and younger were refractory to hypnosis (Gardner & Olness, 1981). These findings are supported by more recent research. Ambrose and Newbold (1968, p. 180) stated that "almost 100 percent of children can be hypnotized." Similarly, other studies have shown that the span from 7.8 years to 11.8 years is the peak of hypnotic susceptibility and that increased imagination is highly, positively correlated with increased responsivity to hypnosis (London & Madsen, 1969).

Gardner and Olness (1981), summarized an extensive review of the literature concerning children's hypnotizability. They noted a number of methodological problems, in particular sampling difficulties, poor assessment measures, induction techniques inappropriate for children, and difficulty in distinguishing simulated hypnosis from actual hypnosis. They concluded that at present little is proven about hypnotic responsiveness in children but that most studies underestimate children's hypnotic abilities, and that using hypnosis with children is very effective in many cases despite the inconsistent findings of research studies. Gardner and Olness recommended that continued use of hypnotic techniques with children, as well as research into the phenomena, should be encouraged.

Psychological and Developmental Characteristics that Improve Hypnotic Responsivity

In order to comprehend why most children are responsive to hypnosis, it is useful to consider certain characteristics typical of children.

Desire for Mastery

Mussen, Conger, and Kagan (1963) identified mastery as a learned motive for children to develop new skills that will allow them to exert control over their environment. This desire to achieve is an important ingredient in children's responsiveness to hypnosis, since the hypnotic technique is something new to learn and is generally taught to give children control over some difficulty which they are experiencing. Thus, children may be told that the therapist is going to teach them a new skill that they can use by themselves to help themselves, thereby capitalizing on their natural desire for mastery. Research findings support the positive correlation between need for achievement and hypnotic responsivity in children (Cooper & London, 1976; Gardner, 1974).

Competitiveness

Closely allied to desire for mastery is competitiveness. Children strive not only to achieve but also to be compared favorably to others who are also trying to achieve (Mussen et al. 1963). While a great deal of competitiveness can be destructive, some competitiveness seems to be necessary for accomplishment. In clinical settings children learn to enter a trance more quickly and easily when they are competing against someone else rather than working alone. Of course, the competition must be structured so that no child feels overwhelmed or defeated by another child's superior ability.

Imagination

Imagination, the process of creating mental images, is extremely important in the use of hypnosis. Olness (1981b) has called imagination the "generic component" of hypnosis. Similarly, Hilgard and Hilgard (1975), Erickson (1958), Udolf (1981), and Gardner (1974) are convinced that hypnotic responsiveness is positively correlated with imagery and the process of imagination. Gardner has delineated several developmental processes in children which probably contribute to their ability to imagine and to respond to hypnosis, including (1) an ability to focus and concentrate on a limited, specific input; (2) a more fluid sense of reality and an ability to shift easily between fantasy and reality; (3) curiosity about and interest in new ideas; and (4) a tendency toward literal and concrete patterns of thought. She believes that these common childhood characteristics contribute significantly to imagination and help to explain why children appear to be very responsive to hypnosis. We would concur in the assessment that imagination is positively correlated with hypnotic responsiveness. However, we would add the caveat that children who do not appear to be very imaginative may still learn to use hypnosis and should not be discouraged from these attempts simply because they are not as fantasy-prone as other children.

Interactions with Adults

From the preceding discussion it would appear that children are indeed quite responsive to hypnosis. However, just as adults are not uniformly responsive to hypnosis, children also vary in their ability to use hypnotic techniques and to respond to hypnotic inductions. Some writers have concentrated on transference and the regressive nature of hypnosis to explain why some children are more responsive than others (Ambrose, 1968; Call, 1976; Krojanker, 1969).

Estabrooks (1962) delineated five dimensions of parent–child interaction that tend to increase the child's responsivity to hypnosis. The first is to gratify the infant's need for dependency so that the child develops a sense of trust from being able to depend upon the parents. The child may then trust the hypnotherapist and accept the hypnotic suggestions. Second, parents develop rules of behavior and disciplinary measures which, when consistent, firm, and based on love convey to a child that the parents are in control and that the child is protected. Accordingly, the child becomes more compliant and familiar with following the suggestions of adults, including those of the hypnotherapist. The third dimension, closely allied to the second, is that parents teach the child to share in and be responsible for performing chores in the house. This helps the child become more conforming with little defiance or hostility. This active conformity is useful in hypnosis as the child makes a conscious effort to engage in the thoughts and/or actions suggested by the hypnotherapist. Fourth, parents who encourage fantasy involvement help their children to maintain vivid imaginations and thus improve responsivity to hypnosis. Finally, the presence of siblings in the home prevents the child from taking on a more adult stance and promotes a primary process or fantasy orientation. This perpetuates imagination, which is a major component in a child's responsivity to hypnosis.

Estabrooks' formulations have been supported by more current research (Hilgard, J.R., 1970; Long, 1969; Nowlis, 1969). Hilgard hypothesized that children who had experienced the parenting patterns suggested by Estabrooks would tend to develop clear identifications and strong egos. Then, when in the hypnotic setting, they would introject the hypnotherapist as a parent and conform to the therapist's authority.

Factors that May Decrease Hypnotic Responsivity

Children may harbor many misconceptions about hypnosis. They often believe that they will be asleep or unconscious, that they will be under the control of the hypnotherapist, or that they will have no recall for events which occur while they are in the trance state. This misinformation may come from parents or other children, but most often seems to be transmitted by television programs and comic books. Even some cartoon shows depict the heroes and heroines under the power of evil professors or aliens because of the use of some hypnotic technique. Generally, explaining hypnosis in an age-appropriate manner will defuse these fears. Sometimes the fact that the children have seen their favorite characters hypnotized actually helps, as they are intrigued by the possibility and are reassured since most children's TV shows and comic books have happy endings.

Negative attitudes about hypnosis held by significant adults in a child's environment may also interfere with the child's responsivity to hypnosis. Many health professionals who work with children harbor the same misconceptions as the laity and therefore do not refer children for hypnotherapy as often as it might be efficacious. Similarly, it has been shown that hypnosis is much more effective when the professional staff working with the patient is supportive (Hartley, 1968). It is clear, then, that the hypnotherapist must ascertain the belief systems concerning hypnosis, of the significant adults, as well as of the children involved, and make attempts to educate whenever necessary.

At times children are fairly refractory to hypnosis, perhaps because of severe emotional or intellectual impairment due to decompensated psychosis, severe mental retardation, extreme pain, or fear. However, the authors have effectively utilized hypnosis in emergency situations, such as at the scene of an automobile accident, where everyone is anxious and somewhat confused. Hypnosis has also been used successfully with a delirious patient (LaBaw, W.L., 1973). Sometimes children are resistant to hypnosis because their symptoms serve an important psychological function for them or because the secondary gain from their symptom is very great. Sometimes they have had, or know someone else who has had, a negative experience with another hypnotherapist. Whatever the cause, it is probably most useful to attempt to discover the cause of the resistance and to work with it before resuming the hypnotherapy.

Tests of Hypnotizability

Before concluding this section on children's responsivity to hypnosis, tests of hypnotizability will be briefly discussed. There are currently two major scales for assessing hypnotizability in children: (1) the Children's Hypnotic Susceptibility Scale, developed by London (1963), and (2) the Stanford Hypnotic Clinical Scale for Children, developed by Morgan and Hilgard (1979). Both of these scales are designed to reveal how responsive a child is to a standardized set of instructions concerning a variety of physical and imaginative tasks. These tasks are designed to reflect or measure certain components of a child's response to hypnosis. There are norms available for London's scale, but no norms are yet available for the newer Stanford Scale for Children. Among hypnotherapists there is controversy about the usefulness of scales of hypnotizability. Many hypnotherapists find them useful, particularly as research tools. Hilgard and Hilgard (1975) believe that subjects who initially are not very responsive to hypnosis can learn to increase their responsiveness and use scales of hypnotizability to measure this. Scales of hypnotizability may be useful in academic or research settings but the authors find little merit to their use in clinical situations, particularly with children. First of all, as previously discussed, most children are responsive to hypnosis, so tests use up valuable time without providing much new information. Second, most of the benefits of the hypnotic state accrue in a fairly light state so it is not important to know if one child is extremely responsive to hypnosis while another is only moderately so. Finally, we have observed children using self-hypnosis very well to achieve their clinical goal, after having failed an hypnotizability scale. We believe that the most efficient way to determine if hypnosis is useful for a child is to attempt a clinical trial, rather than excluding children because they did not perform well on one of the scales. This approach received support at the 25th Annual Meeting of the American Society of Clinical Hypnosis in Denver in 1982; of a panel of eight doctoral-level professionals who work with children, only one uses tests of hypnotizability.

THE PEDIATRIC NURSE AS HYPNOTHERAPIST

As was discussed in the previous section, children tend to be highly responsive to hypnosis and hypnotic techniques. They are also frequent victims of trauma, and suffer from a variety of illnesses and anxiety symptoms known to be amenable to hypnotherapy. Thus, it is extremely important for pediatric nurses to be knowledgeable about hypnosis. This is true even if a nurse does not wish to function as a hypnotherapist, since the literature indicates the efficacy of trance is increased when all persons in the environment are supportive of the technique (LaBaw, 1975; LaBaw, Holton, Tewell, & Eccles, 1975).

We use the term hypnotherapist, rather than hypnotist, throughout this chapter because we believe that hypnosis is most safely and effectively utilized by professionals. While lay hypnotists may sometimes achieve positive results, we are concerned that they may be unable to accurately assess possible physical problems and to make referrals when indicated. Furthermore, we believe that professionals who wish to use hypnotic techniques with children should have specialized education in understanding and working with children above and beyond being skilled in hypnosis. Children present specific and unique problems to any professional—nurse, physician, psychologist, or dentist—and knowledge of normal growth and development and techniques for dealing with children are the minimal tools needed for such work. Therefore, nurses who wish to use hypnosis with children should, in our opinion, have specialized education both in pediatrics and hypnotherapy.

Nurses, in general, use a wide variety of suggestive techniques in their daily interactions with clients. While they may not think of their actions as hypnotic in nature, they utilize many techniques that are commonly employed in hypnotherapy, such as encouragement, distraction, reassurance, calm voice, and soothing touch. Thus, they are already familiar with segments of induction techniques and should be comfortable integrating these tools into an hypnotic induction.

Nurses also tend to spend a large amount of time with clients, engage in a great deal of client education, and may be less associated with painful procedures than other professionals. They are also the most available professionals and the ones who often have the most responsibility for direct, client contact. A skilled professional nurse can utilize these factors to foster a sense of security and trust in the child, and this climate is the most suitable for hypnotherapeutic interventions. Therefore, pediatric nurses are well suited to the role of hypnotherapist and would benefit from learning hypnotherapeutic skills. At the very least, they should be knowledgeable about hypnotherapy in order to facilitate the efforts of colleagues who utilize hypnotherapy.

INDUCTION TECHNIQUES

In order to induce a trance state in a child, the specific technique should be altered to reflect the age of the child. We have found it useful to devise three separate induction routines which cover the span from infancy through adolesence. The ages we have assigned to each technique are somewhat arbitrary and the hypnotherapist should assess the developmental maturity of each child in terms of current emotional and cognitive status and choose the induction technique accordingly. Similarly, the amount of explanation which the nurse should offer the child about the hypnotic process will vary with the age and emotional and physical status of the child.

Infants and Toddlers

The child in the span from birth to three or four years does not have well-developed verbal skills and so will not respond as well to the verbal instructions that are typically utilized to induce a trance state in an adult or older child. However, we believe that infants can and do enter into a state of altered consciousness, as evidenced by clinical results and the trance stare. Since they do not comprehend verbal commands (e.g., "close your eyes"), infants often enter the trance with their eyes open, staring fixedly into space. In this state the therapist may pass a hand in front of the child's eyes and the baby will continue to stare into space, without blinking and without visually tracking the therapist's hand as would be expected of a nonhypnotized, neurologically intact child. Of course, it is essential that the parents and/or primary caretakers are knowledgeable about hypnosis and accept its use with their child.

In order to induce a trance in an infant or very small child, rhythmic stimulation, either tactile, visual, auditory, or a combination of these is utilized. The child may be rocked, patted, rubbed or crooned to, as long as the stimulation is soothing, repetitive, and monotonous. The actual words employed are unimportant, but what seems most effective is a somewhat sing-song, quiet repetition of two or three phrases over and over. The techniques described above are, of course, the ones which have always been employed by parents to soothe or quiet their children in times of distress. The difference in the hypnotic induction is to continue this stimulation beyond the time when the child becomes outwardly calm and extend it to the point that the child enters the altered state of consciousness. The length of time needed to achieve this end is unpredictable and the nurse hypnotherapist will need to assess each child individually. Inducing and maintaining a trance in an infant can be fairly time consuming, and the hypnotherapist may wish to enlist the aid of others to help achieve the desired goals. In hospital settings, volunteers, such as foster grandparents or candy stripers, may be instructed in the rhythmic skills and then monitored periodically by the nurse as they apply the techniques. Similarly, in an outpatient situation, the nurse may teach the parents to utilize these techniques at home. If a child of 2 or 3 years is uncomfortable sitting on the nurse's lap or lying on a couch with the nurse seated nearby, it is sometimes useful to ask a parent to hold the child while the nurse induces the trance. This serves to make the child more comfortable, eases the parent's fears about hypnosis, teaches the parent the rhythmical suggestive techniques, and may also induce a light trance state in the parent. This latter is a desired outcome since anxious infants almost always have anxious parents, and they may also achieve some relief through the trance.

The question might be raised about how often a nurse comes in contact with very young children who are in need of hypnotic intervention. There is no hard, statistical evidence for this query; however, infants and small children do get injured quite often and are subject to a wide variety of anxiety-producing situations. As illustrations of the use of the hypnotic techniques with very young children, two brief case examples follow.

Melissa, age 2 years, suffered from severe trichotillomania (twisting and pulling out her hair). She also ate her hair, and as a result had been hospitalized with intestinal obstructions on two separate occasions. The mother, an extremely anxious woman, was in therapy with a different therapist, but the hope was to find a way to calm Melissa until some of her mother's problems could be resolved. In this case, the mother was simply too tense to assist in the trance induction, so the grandmother's aid was sought. The grandmother held Melissa on her lap while the therapist sat next to her, patting Melissa's back and intoning the repetitive monologue. After several visits Melissa's hair-pulling ceased.

Brandon was a 9-month-old infant who had been severely burned in an accident. He was believed to be mortally injured, although he continued to receive assiduous burn care. He was in severe pain despite the fact that he had been given fairly large doses of morphine. Indeed, he had been given as much as could safely be administered for his body weight, and still he wailed incessantly and loudly. Brandon suffered greatly, and the hospital staff, who were unable to help him, suffered as well. In this case, foster grandparents were enlisted to rock his cradle and a radio, tuned to a quiet, monotonous station, played in the background. These procedures elicited a trance state and kept Brandon quiet and more comfortable for up to 20 minutes at a time. When he began to fuss or cry again, the foster grandparents would resume the rocking. Although he succumbed to his burns, these hypnotic techniques allowed him to die more comfortably.

Toddlers and Preadolescents

Children from 3 to 11 or 12 years of age tend to be sociable, to enjoy games, and to follow directions. These traits may be utilized to induce a trance state. When working with children in this age group it is useful to describe the trance induction as a relaxing game that you are going to teach them in order to help them control whatever their symptoms might be. Of course, the hypnotherapist will need to alter the amount of information and explanation about this relaxing game and its purpose based on the individual child's developmental stage and verbal ability. When formulating an induction routine to use with children, it is most efficient and useful to use words which are easily understood by even very young children. Thus, the explanation will not need to be changed with each child. This allows the hypnotherapist to work with groups made up of children of a variety of ages and also maintain a smoother technique. To this end, these authors tend to use such words as "easy," "rested," and "relaxed."

The relaxing game is merely a variation of the child's game, "Simon Says," called "Doctor Says" or "Nurse Says" (LaBaw, 1973). In this game, the child performs various actions as directed but only obeys those commands prefaced by "Doctor says. . . ." After several instructions have been offered, the command "Doctor says to close your eyes" is given and the monologue ensues. As the child focuses on the sound of the therapist's voice, rather than the content, and begins to enter the trance state, the use of the phrase "Doctor says. . . ." may be discontinued. A variation of this relaxing game may be introduced, in which idyllic imagery is utilized to lengthen the trance. In this case, after the child is in a hypnoidal state he or she is directed to imagine a pleasant, tranquil scene such as a beach, a mountain lake, or forest. The setting should be one with which the child has experience and one about which there are pleasant associations. The therapist then describes the scene, stressing the most pleasant, soothing aspects, while maintaining a rhythmical, monotonous style of delivery. The therapist may allow the child to linger in this pleasant fantasy by giving the child permission to persist in the fantasy as long as he or she chooses, at which time, the therapist may leave or simply remain quiet until the child arouses. This technique of extending the trance is especially useful with children in pain, as they can be relatively free of discomfort or at least more comfortable while they remain in the trance state. They may also be instructed to maintain the trance until they fall asleep. Again, this is especially useful with children who have significant pain, who often have a great deal of difficulty falling asleep without analgesics or hypnotic chemicals.

When teaching children this relaxing game, it is often useful to take advantage of their natural competitiveness as well as the normal contagion of the trance state. Thus, two or more children can play the game at the same time and, as they do so, try to outperform one another. The result of this competition is that the children tend to enter the trance more quickly and easily. If other children are not available, the participation of the parents or hospital personnel may be enlisted. The therapist may also choose to use toys such as dolls or stuffed animals. With younger children, it is often helpful to use a toy (e.g., a teddy bear) that is not very good at the game and makes mistakes and over which the child can easily triumph. For older children, the toy, a crafty crow for example, needs to be smarter and make fewer mistakes in order to fuel the competition. However, in all cases, the child should feel that, with some effort, he or she can win the game.

For children past the toddler stage, the emphasis is on self-hypnosis. These children are instructed, both in and out of the trance state, that they may play the relaxing game or reexperience the idyllic scene simply by closing their eyes and remembering the sound of the therapist's voice. With experience, practice and time, most 4 and 5 year olds can learn to self-induce the trance state and apply it in a somewhat systematic fashion. Some of these children, particularly the younger ones, may require some help from their parents, such as reminders to practice their relaxing game, keeping siblings away, or decreasing extraneous noises. Learning self-induction allows the children to become independent of the therapist and provides a tool that they can use for themselves to help them feel more comfortable in any situation. Thus, these children feel more confident, competent, and in control.

Adolescents

While some pre-adolescents and early adolescents may persist in the more compliant postures of the typical latency-age child, most are more challenging and rebellious and thus require somewhat of a different approach. Also, they may harbor some of the same common misconceptions about hypnosis that many adults have and which contribute to resistance to hypnosis. Therefore, it is probably best to approach these young people in a more adult manner, explaining as much as possible about what hypnosis is and how it may be able to help them. It is often useful to appeal to their scientific curiosity and to stress that this technique is *their* tool to use for themselves. It is important to note, however, that it is not very difficult to establish rapport and elicit the cooperation of an adolescent, or anyone else for that matter, to use hypnosis. This is because there is usually a specific symptom present that the client would like to be rid of and therefore he or she is very motivated to proceed and willing to accept the hypnotherapist's instructions. This cooperation is especially apparent when the symptom involved is pain.

Once rapport is established with an adolescent and any questions or concerns have been addressed, the trance induction may proceed by the technique normally utilized by the therapist. The authors use a fairly straightforward, monotonous monologue, but vary the routine by including idyllic imagery or some progressive relaxation steps. These variations are introduced either to prolong the experience or to improve response if the child seems to be having trouble achieving the trance state. Thus, the authors work with older children and adolescents in a manner similar to that used with adults.

Differences Between Children's and Adults' Responses to Hypnosis

Children, unlike adults, usually do not have any preconceived idea about how people behave when hypnotized. Therefore, while adults may sit or lie quite still, children often move about. They may rock or sway, swing their legs, tap their fingers, or even flap their arms as if they had wings. Some children relinquish these behaviors either as they become more deeply relaxed or as they become more accustomed to the hypnotic induction, while other children persist in these behaviors. In any case, it is probably best if the therapist ignores these behaviors, unless they are too disruptive or appear designed to resist the induction, and simply continues the hypnotic routine. Additionally, children are often very amused by the process of hypnotic induction and may smile or laugh out loud when the therapist begins the monologue. It is often easiest to circumvent this behavior by predicting for the child that he or she may be amused by the process or may think the therapist sounds funny and that this is all right, as long as the child keeps his or her eyes comfortably closed and continues to listen to the therapist's voice. Similarly, if the child does laugh during the induction, the therapist may simply accept that the child finds it amusing and repeat the instructions stated above. Children also will often open one or both eyes to check on what the therapist, or anyone else in the room, is doing. In this case, the therapist may simply tell the child to shut his or her eyes again and to keep them comfortably closed and continue with the induction.

As stated in an earlier section of this chapter, it is very important to obtain informed consent for the use of hypnosis from the child's guardians. However, despite thorough explanations about the nature of hypnosis, many parents will persist in some unrealistic fears or expectations about the trance state. One easy way to allay these concerns is to invite the parents or guardians to observe a trance session after the child has become adept at entering the altered state of consciousness. This serves to reassure the parents that the therapist is doing no more or less than that which was described to them. This also gives the child a chance to perform for the parents, to display the new skill, and to accept the praise of the therapist in the presence of the parents. Such a process may improve the child's feelings of self-worth, increase allegiance to the technique, and strengthen determination to practice the trance.

Children in trance may experience the same physiological changes and other sensations that adults report about their trance experience. They may state that they feel relaxed or more comfortable or they may describe the warmth that accompanies vasodilation. If they are attached to the appropriate measuring devices, it is possible to demonstrate that the blood pressure and heart rate also decrease. The therapist may also observe that respiratory patterns change as oxygen consumption decreases in the altered state and that many children have the eyelid flutter reflex typical of the hypnoidal state. Additionally, children often experience paresthesias such as numbness, tingling, heaviness, lightness, and/or feelings of dissociation. Some children, as some adults, are bothered or frightened by dissociative feelings. If, after some reassurance, dissociative feelings continue to interfere, the therapist may instruct children to open their eyes while in the trance and reassure themselves that body integrity is maintained and then to close their eyes again. Following this procedure once or twice usually mitigates most concerns. Conversely, paresthesias may also be employed as reinforcers for practicing the trance technique, e.g., one 8-year-old boy likened his strong dissociative feeling to the feeling of weightlessness in space. Thereafter, he eagerly practiced his "space walk" and boasted to his friends that he knew what it would feel like to be an astronaut!

CLINICAL APPLICATIONS

Hypnosis is, at the very least, a useful adjunct in the treatment of problems in which anxiety is a mediator, and at times hypnosis is a primary means of treatment. The anxiolytic property of the trance state is the most important therapeutic aspect of hypnosis. Therefore, we believe that inducing the trance state is of primary concern and that any suggestions which are offered once the hypnotic state has been induced are of secondary importance. This position is supported by the fact that preverbal children achieve desired effects from the trance state, as well as by the fact that many persons successfully apply the hypnotic technique to problems other than those for which they learned it and for which they received no specific suggestions. This is not to say that we do not utilize a wide variety of suggestions, but that our main concern is induction of the trance state. When suggestions are used, care should be taken to individualize the suggestions. This is particularly important when working with children and must take into account the cognitive development of the child, especially verbal abilities, cultural idiosyncrasies, and emotional reactions. Additionally, it must be remembered that children are often very literal and concrete in their thinking and respond to suggestions in a similar manner.

The following pages will focus on a variety of problems for which we have found hypnosis to be a useful, therapeutic tool.

Habit Disorders

Many childhood habits may be amenable to treatment with hypnosis. Although habits are often established for some emotional reason, most often for anxiety reduction, some seem to evolve from a learning paradigm and to be strengthened by simple repetition in the face of similar stimuli. It is important to determine what, if any, emotional attachment the child may have to the symptom and what secondary gains may be present. If there are important familial interactions that center around the child and/or the symptom, some form of family intervention may need to occur either prior to or concurrently with the attempt to remove the symptom. Similarly, the hypnotherapist should assess the child's motivation to relinquish the symptom. Sometimes, the person who experiences distress concerning the symptom is the parent, not the child. However, most school-age children are very eager to give up annoying habits. They often feel embarrassed by their habits and anticipate feeling less conspicuous when they cease nail biting, bedwetting, or other symptoms. If after three to five sessions the child has not learned the self-hypnotic technique, is not practicing, or has not experienced diminution of the symptom, it is necessary to explore the nature of the child's resistance and seek a resolution. Such resistance might be due to a lack of trust in or rapport with the hypnotherapist, the child's unresolved conscious or unconscious fears about hypnosis, parental resistance to the change, or the child's emotional need to maintain the symptom. Sometimes, the child is simply not sufficiently motivated to relinquish the symptom and, in this case, attempts to remove the symptom should cease until such time as the child is ready to expend the necessary effort.

Parents are often concerned about the possibility of symptom substitution. That is, they have heard of people who give up a fairly innocuous symptom such as nail biting only to replace it with a worse symptom such as bedwetting. In our experience, this has not occurred, nor are we aware of any documented cases in the literature. It seems as though children are either glad to be rid of their symptom or, if they still need or want it for some reason, simply maintain it. There is really no need for them to give up one symptom only to replace it with another. From a dynamic perspective, it is possible to think of this process as a net psychic gain rather than a loss which needs to be corrected. In other words, an eneuretic child who learns hypnosis to stop wetting the bed *gains* a tool to control the eneurisis rather than losing the symptom.

Nail Biting, Thumb Sucking, Trichotillomania

These habits are fairly common, not generally associated with any physical causes, and probably result from anxiety. Initially, we try to ascertain the source of the child's anxiety, but seldom find any specific cause. In general, children with these symptoms tend to worry about many things, to strive for achievement, and to be somewhat self-critical. They function with a constant level of fairly high anxiety, which is largely unrelated to external events. Occasionally, it is possible to determine some specific environmental or emotional stressor which is generating the anxiety and then the child and the family are referred for the appropriate therapeutic intervention, which may or may not include hypnotherapy. However, most children who suffer from one of these symptoms do not know the source of their anxiety, claim to be unaware of their behavior when engaging in it, and want to control it because it is embarrassing. While trichotillomania is not as common as the other two habits addressed in this section— Horne (1977) discovered only a few cases in the literature—we have recently received several referrals for this problem. These have included some fairly unusual instances of hair pulling; a 15-year-old male who had been pulling out his eyelashes for five years and was, as a result, suffering from chronic eye irritation, and an adolescent female who was pulling out her pubic hair.

These disorders tend to be very amenable to hypnotherapy as the trance destroys the anxiety which propels the habit, provides the child with an alternative behavior and, through direct suggestion, reinforces the child's desire to control the behavior. The child is told in the trance state, "You will be aware of any urge to pull your hair (bite your nails, suck your thumb, etc.) and will be able to control it. You will be aware any time your hand goes to your mouth (or hair). The more often you use this state of relaxation, the less often you will find yourself pulling your hair (putting your hand to your mouth, etc.)"

The child is instructed to practice self-hypnosis three times a day and at any other time he or she feels anxious, feels the desire to engage in the unwanted behavior, or anticipates being in a situation that might produce anxiety. Sometimes children who are very imaginative enjoy adding their own images to the trance routine, e.g. imagining pretty, healthy hair or more attractive hands, and this is encouraged. In our experience, five appointments—two one week, two the following week and one approximately one month later as a follow-up and reinforcer—are usually sufficient to control these habits. Of course, if a child is motivated and determined but has not achieved the desired success, we add one or two appointments until the goal is reached.

Eneuresis

Eneuresis is the involuntary voiding of urine occurring after an age at which continence is expected and which is not due to any physiological cause. This problem is most common at night (nocturnal) but may also occur during the day (diurnal) or at both times. Eneuresis is called primary if there has been a lack of urinary continence for one year, and secondary if it occurs following at least one year of urinary continence (American Psychiatric Association, 1980). According to Cohen (1975), this is a very common problem which has occurred in 20 million Americans over the age of 5 years.

Since eneuresis may be due to a wide variety of structural defects and/or illnesses such as diabetes, seizures, urinary tract infections, neurological disorders, and possibly some allergies, it is extremely important that children referred for hypnotherapy for eneuresis have a thorough physical examination first. With secondary eneuresis, it is also important to determine if the child has experienced any unusual stresses or significant changes in family structure or lifestyle which might have precipitated the symptom.

In treating eneuresis we combine behavioral techniques with hypnotherapy and sometimes also utilize a course of imipramine. The children and their parents are instructed to allow the children to take care of changing beds and washing their own sheets, with some parental help if the child is very young. The parents are also told to be as uninvolved as possible and to treat any accidents in a very neutral, matter-of-fact manner. The children are told to restrict fluids prior to bedtime.

Most eneuretic children feel embarrassed and ashamed of their symptom and are eager to resolve the problem so that they can join their peers at camps or can sleep over at friends' houses. The hypnotherapist can help these children feel more comfortable by being accepting of the problem, recognizing that the children are not willfully urinating, reinforcing the belief that they can learn to control the problem, and utilizing the same terminology for urinating as the families use. This last technique seems to be especially important with younger children, who appear relieved when the hypnotherapist uses familiar terms. To this end it is useful to ask the parents, prior to the first visit, what terms are utilized for urination and use these terms throughout.

Hypnotherapy for eneuresis proceeds in the same manner as for other problems. The children are initially instructed in the use of self-hypnosis and then specific suggestions for their problem are introduced. They are told that they will be aware of the urge to urinate even if they are asleep and that they will get up and urinate in the toilet; that they will enjoy the good, pleasant feeling of a dry bed; that they will feel very good about themselves for gaining this control. The children are then instructed to practice self-hypnosis at least three times a day and to use it to help themselves to fall asleep at night and that this will reinforce their desire and ability to stay dry. In our experience, these techniques are highly effective in the treatment of eneuresis and most children can learn to control this symptom in four to six visits. Sometimes, children will experience a recurrence of eneuretic symptoms after being dry for a period of time. In this case, a review of self-hypnosis generally allows a quick return to continence.

Encopresis

Encopresis is the passing of feces at inappropriate times (as defined by the child's culture), occurring after an age at which bowel control is expected, and not due to any physiological disorder. Encopresis is called primary if it occurs after the age of 4 and there has not been a one-year period of fecal continence. Secondary encopresis is used to refer to encopresis that follows at least one year of fecal continence (APA, 1980).

In general, encopresis is less common and more often due to physiological causes than is eneuresis. Many times encopresis signifies constipation with fecal material leaking around a blockage. Therefore it is crucial that a child with encopresis receive a thorough physical examination. If constipation or any other physiological disorder is diagnosed, it should be treated by dietary, behavioral and/or pharamocological techniques rather than with hypnotherapy.

If all physiological causes have been ruled out, the hypnotherapist should proceed by taking a detailed history from the parents about the child's stool habits, the child's reaction to toilet training attempts, any significant changes in the child's life, and parental reactions to the their child's soiling. With primary encopretic children, in particular, it is important to determine their feelings about sitting on the toilet. This is because fears about the toilet, which may have begun in infancy, can lead to a resistance to using the toilet as the child grows older. The word or words that the child uses to describe bowel movements should also be ascertained by the therapist and utilized from the first session.

In treating encopresis, we give the responsibility for staying clean to the children. They are instructed to clean themselves and their underclothing, as necessary, and to sit on the toilet for 10 to 15 minutes either after breakfast or after dinner (the children should choose which of these times they prefer and then adhere to that schedule). The parents are told to respond to accidents in a neutral manner and to allow their children to take responsibility for cleaning themselves. The children are then taught self-hypnosis and specific suggestions for bowel control are introduced. The children are told that they will recognize the feeling of needing to defecate; that they will defecate in a toilet; that they will be able to control sphincter muscles until they are able to reach a toilet; that they will be able to relax once they are seated on a toilet; that they will enjoy being clean and that they will feel very good about themselves for achieving this control. They are also instructed to practice the self-hypnosis at least three times a day, including while they are seated on the toilet for the required time.

In our experience, encopresis is more difficult to treat than eneuresis. We may need six or eight appointments to obtain positive results. These children often seem to have other significant emotional problems which also need therapy. Family therapy, concurrent with hypnotherapy, is sometimes needed to achieve complete control. Additionally, children with chronic encopresis may experience some loss of muscle tone in the anal sphincter and continue some leaking of fecal material even when defecating regularly in the toilet.

Situational Disorders

Children who suffer from difficulties which will be discussed in this section tend to be very anxious and concerned about their specific problems. Unlike habits, of which most children claim to be unaware, children who suffer from situational disorders can usually describe those situations that cause them significant problems. Examples of situational disorders include performance anxieties, phobic disorders, and sleep disorders.

Performance Anxieties

Anxiety may significantly interfere with children's abilities to perform in a variety of settings. Children who compete in athletics may discover that they perform very well during practice but experience many difficulties and make many errors in actual competition. Similarly, children may have a great deal of trouble performing well on school tests or reciting in class. They may have studied diligently, yet when required to reproduce learned material they may have difficulty remembering information or expressing what they know in a logical, cogent fashion. They may blush or stammer when called on in class or forget their lines in a school play. All of these are examples of performance anxiety and are primary indicators for the use of hypnotherapy.

In order to alleviate performance anxiety, children should be taught self-hypnosis, told that they can recapture this relaxed feeling in the performance situation, and told that staying relaxed will allow them to perform to the best of their ability. It is also useful to have them imagine themselves successfully performing the activity. They should practice the trance often in nonstressful settings, and then use it before and even during the actual performance. It is useful to problem-solve with children about how they can use self-hypnosis in the particular performance setting which is difficult for them. For example, ski racers can be told to enter the trance state at the top of the hill, leaning on their ski poles while waiting to maneuver into the starting gate. Students can rest their heads on their hands and trance before beginning an exam or at any time they feel themselves becoming anxious or having difficulty recalling material. If there are no other options, children can be instructed to go to a restroom and trance while sitting on the commode.

In our experience, almost all performance anxieties may be quickly eliminated in three or four sessions with the use of hypnotherapy. If, after a clinical trial of hypnotherapy, a high level of anxiety remains, further exploration of the psychological implications of the activity or the individual's investment in it is indicated.

Phobic Disorders

Phobias are characterized by an extreme, irrational fear of a specific object, activity, or situation which causes children to limit or organize their life in such a way as to avoid the feared object, activity, or situation. Although phobias are fairly easily resolved through hypnotherapy, many parents assume that children who have a phobia are merely going through a "stage" and will outgrow it. This is sometimes the case, but more often phobic children become phobic adults. Therefore, it probably makes sense to treat phobias promptly, before they become entrenched.

We use a combination of hypnotherapy and systematic desensitization to treat phobias, although we proceed through the desensitization more rapidly than is typical of some behaviorial models. We use either imagery or in vivo desensitization, depending upon the phobic stimulus. For example, if the phobia is a fear of heights (acrophobia) we teach the child self-hypnosis and then, while the child remains in the trance state, we ride up and down the elevator in our office building. If the phobic reaction is to some stimulus that cannot be easily replicated in the office, we ask the child to think of some aspect of the stimulus which is least frightening and then proceed through a brief hierarchy. We suggest that the child can remain relaxed and feel pleasant, calm, and in control in the presence of the feared stimulus. We stress feelings of mastery and confidence and suggest that the child can recapture these feelings anytime he or she enters the trance state or is exposed to the phobic situation. The child is asked to practice this at home, utilizing self-hypnosis and imagining being calm and in control while encountering the feared situation.

Hypnotherapy tends to resolve phobias, if the children are diligent in their practice, within 4 to 6 appointments. If there is little or no progress in this time span, the therapist should more closely examine the psychological implications of the phobia and the familial interaction around the phobia. Some children who appear phobic are merely copying parental behavior toward a specific situation and receive parental support for their avoidance behavior. On the other hand, the phobia may be an overt manifestation of some significant personality disturbance and, in this case, the child should be referred for more extensive psychological therapy.

Sleep Disorders

Insomnia, fear of going to sleep, nightmares, sleepwalking, nocturnal bruxism (grinding of the teeth), and nocturnal clenching of the jaw are all symptoms which we have found to be amenable to hypnotherapy. Children with any of these symptoms are taught a basic self-induction and instructed to practice three times a day. They are also told to trance at night, in bed, until they fall asleep, that using the trance in this manner will allow them to sleep easily throughout the night, and if they waken during the night, they may use the self-hypnosis to return quickly and easily to a pleasant, easy state of sleep. They are also instructed to remain in their bed, with all of their muscles soft, relaxed, and comfortable. Again, four appointments followed by a month of practicing and a final appointment seem to be very effective for these problems.

Physical Disorders

In addition to the disorders for which hypnotherapy is a primary means of treatment, there are also many pediatric medical problems for which it is an important adjunctive treatment. In these cases the basic medical problems are treated by a variety of medical means and the trance is used to modify the severity of the problems or to alleviate one or more of the symptoms associated with the physical disorder. The exception to this may be migraine headaches, which often appear to be cured by using hypnotherapy alone.

In general, children who suffer from physical maladies, whether chronic or immediate, view themselves as different and not as "good" as other children. They may believe that their physical problem is punishment for some imagined guilt or that they will constantly have to strive to deserve to live and be cared for by others. These factors tend to make them feel helpless, inadequate, and chronically anxious. At times, these feelings may be so strong that hypnotherapy is of limited value until their psychological status is improved. However, for most of these children, hypnotherapy is a tool which they can use for themselves not only to ameliorate their physical symptoms but also to enhance their feelings of competency, mastery, and self-worth. Since they are the ones who wield the tool, they feel more in control and more confident.

Burns

Burned children present a myriad of complex physical and emotional difficulties. In addition to shock, tissue damage, pain, infection, and stress ulcers, they are prone to severe depression, guilt fantasies, fear, and regression. While there is, of course, no substitute for the assiduous care provided by professionals skilled in the care of burns, some aspects of this trauma, namely, regressive soiling and lack of food and fluid intake, are best treated by hypnotherapy. Additionally, hypnotherapy may also be utilized to decrease discomfort, either alone or in conjunction with analgesics, and thereby make treatment procedures less stressful and promote rest and healing.

The emotional regression which occurs following any severe trauma is especially significant in burned children. These children have large open areas, denuded of skin, and are thus very susceptible to infection. Traumatic eneuresis and encopresis, which are frequent concomitants of emotional regression, can lead to fatal infections if intestinal pathogens invade the burned areas. Infection can also delay skin-grafting procedures and impede healing. Even the most assiduous nursing care cannot prevent these children from being exposed to the bacteria from their own bowels, as they often leak fecal material and urine fairly consistently. LaBaw (1973) used hypnosis with a series of 23 severely burned children and stated that traumatic eneuresis and encopresis "which otherwise can persist for weeks, can usually be stopped in days" using hypnotherapy. The procedure for this is the same as for nontraumatic soiling; these children are encouraged to stay dry and clean, to call for assistance when they have to defecate or urinate, and to feel very good about themselves for staying clean and dry.

Another concomitant of regression and depression which is especially harmful to burn victims is anorexia. At a time when food and fluid need is highest to replenish the fluid which exudes from the injured tissues and to fuel the restoration and healing process, burned children have little appetite. This indifference to oral intake can be quickly reversed through hypnotherapy. The suggestions offered are that the child will feel hungry and thirsty, that food will taste good, and that when the nurse brings something to drink he or she will drink it all, enjoying how good it tastes.

Alleviation of pain, both from the burns themselves, as well as from necessary procedures such as debridement, is another indication for the use of hypnotherapy in the management of burned children. Hypnosis has been shown to be an effective means of diminishing, or even abolishing, discomfort from a variety of causes, including burns (LaBaw, 1973; Wakeman & Kaplan, 1978). Sometimes a combination of hypnotherapy and chemical analgesia is most successful, but often children can remain comfortable throughout very painful procedures using only hypnosis. Whichever approach is used, children using self-hypnosis are less sedated, less fearful of painful procedures, more cooperative, and feel more confident and more in control. The suggestions utilized for pain relief are that the children can feel more comfortable and better as they use the trance, that they can be better able to tolerate any slight discomfort which might remain, and that any feeling of discomfort will be a signal to them to become even more relaxed. At no time are they promised that they will feel no discomfort since any pain sensation or even a feeling of pressure may then be interpreted as pain and evidence that the trance is not effective.

One further possibility for the use of hypnosis with burned children is in the area of limiting burn damage and facilitating healing. Although there are no data available as yet to support this, Gardner and Olness (1981) believe that children can use hypnotherapy to improve healing, based on other evidence of the effect of hypnotherapy on dermatological problems and vascular control. Other researchers are attempting to limit the depth of burns by using hypnotherapy in the emergency room. They hope that significant deep tissue damage may be limited by hypnotherapy. Again, there are no data available on the efficacy of these techniques.

Terminal Illness

There are many published reports concerning the effectiveness of hypnotherapy with terminally ill children. Many of these are anecdotal in nature and based only on a small number of clients. However, the sheer number of cases reported in the literature and our own experience convince us that hypnotherapy is a useful adjunct in the treatment of many physiological and psychological symptoms which accompany terminal illness.

Children with life-threatening illnesses are prone to regression and depression, which lead to anorexia. This loss of appetite is worsened by the toxic effect of some treatments such as chemotherapy and radiation therapy. These children, whose nutritional status is already compromised by their psychological state, often become nauseous from treatments and refrain from eating or vomit what they do ingest. Sometimes they even engage in anticipatory emesis (vomiting prior to receiving treatments). Thus, at a time when the nutritional need is very high, children tend to eat and drink even less than normally and compromise their physical status even more. LaBaw et al. (1975) used hypnotherapy with 27 terminally ill children and found that they could increase food and fluid intake, decrease vomiting, and stop anticipatory vomiting. Olness (1981a) taught self-hypnosis to 21 children, with the result that anorexia and nausea decreased. The procedures used to treat anorexia in these children are the same as that described for burn victims. We also add the suggestions that the children will be able to retain what they eat and that their stomachs will feel easier and better as they use the trance.

Children who are terminally ill suffer discomfort from their basic illnesses as well as from diagnostic and treatment procedures. Hypnotherapy has been shown to be useful with pain in this client population (LaBaw et al., 1975; Olness, 1981a). We use the procedures outlined in the previous discussion on pain in burned children. In our experience, children who utilize self-hypnosis are far calmer during all procedures and experience less discomfort than children who do not have this tool. In fact, LaBaw (1975) described a 7-year-old boy who used only self-hypnosis as anesthesia for sternal bone marrow aspiration.

The idea of using hypnotherapy and imagery to directly affect the course of a terminal illness has garnered more interest in the past few years. As evidence accumulates that implicates psychological factors in the etiology of some terminal illnesses, the possibility that psychological factors could be mobilized to treat these illnesses is also raised. While we know of no data supporting this position, we believe that it is logical and know that hypnotherapy does not have harmful effects for the terminally ill. Thus, when we are asked to use hypnotherapy and imagery to modify a terminal illness we explain our position to the client and family, stating that there is no evidence of its effectiveness nor any reason not to believe it is beneficial. We also explain that there are other positive effects to be gained from self-hypnosis, e.g., less anxiety, easier sleep, less pain, and better nutrition. We also require these patients to remain on their medical regime and to continue with more traditional treatments.

The process of using hypnotherapy and imagery to affect terminal illness is fairly simple. We ask the clients how they visualize their disease-fighting process and then teach them self-hypnosis. We ask them, in the trance state, to visualize these processes destroying the illness and to focus on feeling better, visualizing themselves as healthy and active. The visual imagery need have nothing to do with actual physiology; what is important is that the children are able to visualize a clear image. Some of the images we have heard clients use are "an army of Pac-men gobbling up the bad stuff," "a good army fighting a bad army," and "thousands of little cells swarming all over the tumor like ants on a sugar cube, eating it up."

Some of the children with whom we have used hypnosis and imagery have died and some continue to progress quite well. We continue to use imagery and self-hypnosis with terminally ill children even though we cannot prove that it directly affects the course of the illness, because it may be effective in this way. It also has no harmful effects and many positive ones, and it helps to provide the children with some feelings of control, mastery, and hope.

Hemophilia

Hemophilia is an inherited illness in which there is a lack of clotting factor VIII. There are also other bleeding disorders similar to hemophilia, such as factor VII or factor IX deficiencies. All of these disorders are characterized by spontaneous bleeding as well as increased bleeding from trauma. These spontaneous bleeds seem to occur most often into joints, particularly elbows and knees, but can occur in body cavities or internal organs. Bleeds are treated by intravenous infusion of the specific clotting factor which is deficient. The severity of this disorder is determined by the relative lack of clotting factor; thus a child with very little clotting factor will have a more severe form of the disorder than a child whose clotting factor is only slightly below the normal level. The illness is carried by mothers, who do not manifest the disease but who pass the illness on to their sons. Each son of a carrier mother has a 50-50 chance of inheriting the disorder and each daughter, a 50-50 chance of becoming a carrier. Hemophilia is a disease of males and only affects females in rare genetic interactions.

Hypnotherapy cannot, of course, change the genetic structure which causes hemophilia, but it can alter some of the manifestations of the disorder.

Steinhausen (1975) suggested that hemophilia is a good example of how a disease process can be adversely affected by a negative psychological state, namely anxiety. Other researchers such as Agle (1964) and Mattsson and Gross (1966) offered support for the theory that stress could influence both the severity and frequency of bleeds. Spencer (1971) noted a coincidence of increased frequency of spontaneous bleeds and overprotective parents. Browne, Mally, and Kane (1960) found a high correlation between spontaneous bleeds and times of conflict in 28 subjects studied over an eight-month period. Therefore, since stress increases spontaneous bleeds, it is likely that the anxiolytic effect of hypnotherapy can reduce the number of bleeds.

Wallace LaBaw (1970, 1975) conducted a controlled study which supports the tenet that a positive psychological state can decrease bleeding in hemophiliacs. Twenty subjects were randomly assigned to a control or an experimental group, with the experimental group learning self-hypnosis but in other respects receiving the same treatment as the control group. The unit of measurement was the amount of transfusion product used. After 40 months the experimental group had used statistically significant less blood and blood products than the control group.

In 1975, Jeanine LaBaw (LaBaw & LaBaw, 1977) developed the idea of summer camps as a medium for teaching self-hypnosis as well as providing typical camp experiences to raise self-esteem and increase confidence and mastery in hemophilic children. This camp continues to function under the auspices of the University of Colorado Health Sciences Center and seems to be achieving its goals.

In our experience, most hemophiliacs who have learned hypnotherapy report increased feelings of well-being and decreased bleeding episodes. While there is no proof of the mechanism by which trance decreases bleeding, the current assumption is that stress interferes with platelet aggregation. For hemophiliacs, who already have the tendency to bleed, this added burden or faulty platelet aggregation increases the problem and contributes to bleeding episodes. LaBaw's techniques have been emulated elsewhere, and there is a current attempt to replicate LaBaw's techniques with hemophiliacs from Johns Hopkins.

The technique we employ with hemophiliacs is similar to that described for other client groups. A group format seems especially useful with this client population. The children learn by imitating one another and the relaxed state seems to be fairly contagious. Parents often observe the session or try to participate. This is useful since the anxiety of parents is often communicated to their children. We remind the boys, in trance, that they will remain alert to any problems with their bleeding disorder and seek appropriate medical treatment, that they should use trance preventively several times a day and at any time they find themselves feeling anxious, and that staying relaxed will allow them to bleed less often and less severely. We also remind them that they may use the trance to deal with the discomfort of the actual bleed, which can be excruciating, since the joint capsule, already full of synovial fluid, is flooded with blood and the pressure may be intense. Similarly, they may modify the discomfort of chronic arthritis, which often results in hemophiliacs from joint deterioration.

One other aspect of hemophilia which should be mentioned at this time is the fact that hemophiliacs have been designated at risk for Acquired Immune Deficiency Syndrome (AIDS). It is assumed, but not proven, that AIDS is somehow transmitted through transfusion products. Until such time as the mechanism for the transmission of AIDS can be fully discovered, hematologists appear to be recommending that hemophiliacs continue to treat bleeds with transfusions but to avoid unnecessary transfusions. Therefore, it seems urgent that more hemophiliacs attempt to decrease bleeds through the use of self-hypnosis in order to decrease their need for transfusions. Similarly, since stress increases bleeds, a hemophiliac's increased anxiety and worry about contracting AIDS could be assuaged through the use of self-hypnosis.

Asthma

Asthma is a respiratory disorder in which there is obstruction of the lower respiratory tract with the result that breathing becomes labored and characterized by wheezing. In the past, professionals have disagreed about whether or not asthmatic attacks were triggered by exposure to some element in the physical environment or if they were psychologically induced. More current information seems to indicate that one type of asthma has more of an external physiological trigger, while another type may occur due to factors internal to the patient, including anxiety. Even if the asthma attack is initially triggered by a purely physical stimulus, difficulty in breathing results in severe anxiety and even further bronchoconstriction. Cohen, Goodenough, and Witkin (1975) have demonstrated that even in normal subjects anxiety changes the respiratory cycle and results in increased expiratory time, which is characteristic of asthma. Other studies and observations have indicated that suggestion and learned responses can also trigger an asthmatic attack (Kahn, Staerk, & Bonk, 1974). Indeed, Kahn (1973) has claimed that "as high as 50 percent (of asthma) is essentially nonallergic and (of the type) in which emotions rank high among precipitants."

While the exact effect of psychological factors in the etiology of asthma is yet to be completely elucidated, it seems clear that anxiety can have a deleterious effect. Therefore, it is also logical to assume that hypnotherapy and direct suggestion could positively alter the asthmatic response. Collison (1975) used hypnotherapy with 121 asthmatic clients and reported that 21 percent became free of asthma, 33 percent decreased the frequency and severity of their attacks, and 46 percent had little or no response but indicated a subjective increase in feelings of well-being. In our experience, self-hypnosis has been a very useful adjunct in the treatment of asthma, to prevent, abort, or decrease the severity of an attack. However, one caveat must be added: asthmatic children are often the center of a great deal of attention within their families. While this may be true of children with any chronic illness, it seems especially the case with asthmatic children, possibly because of the life-threatening nature of respiratory problems. Whatever the reason, it is important for the hypnotherapist to assess the functions that the asthma may serve within the family and attempt to defuse the emotional responses of the family members. Sometimes this may be achieved by having the child take more responsibility for managing the asthmatic condition, but other times more intensive family therapy is indicated.

The procedure for using hypnotherapy with asthma is fairly simple and similar to that which has been previously described. The children are taught self-hypnosis and told to use the technique several times a day and at the first sign of any respiratory distress. The suggestion is made that using the trance will relax the muscles surrounding the bronchial tree and allow air to move in and out, smoothly and easily. Sometimes it is useful to draw a picture of the bronchial tree and show the children where the difficulty occurs and ask them to imagine loosening the constriction and breathing more easily. Most children find their asthma to be very physically limiting, are motivated to learn the trance, and do so in three to four sessions.

Headaches

Some common types of headaches in the pediatric population are either migraine headaches due to vascular changes or tension headaches due to muscle contractions. However, headaches may also be the presenting symptom of a wide array of physiological disorders. It is therefore important to rule out physical causes before attempting to treat headaches with hypnotherapy. However, even if the headache is not psychogenic, self-hypnosis may be used to decrease discomfort until the physiological cause can be treated.

Treatment of headaches with self-hypnosis instead of with pharmacological agents is especially important in a pediatric population. Olness and McDonald (1981) state that the use of drugs to treat these headaches has resulted in inadequate clinical results, undesirable side effects, concern that there is a correlation between prescribed psychoactive drugs and the subsequent use of illicit drugs in adolescents, and a fear that the use of drugs to deal with stress as a child leads to inadequate coping skills as an adult. Therefore, hypnotic techniques, which stress mastery, self-control, and mobilization of innate capabilities, are an excellent alternative.

Children are often unaware of the stressors in their environment, and it is usually not necessary to spend a great deal of time trying to determine what they are. We teach children self-hypnosis and suggest that they may use the trance both to become more aware of their unconscious stress and to let that stress flow out of their minds. We suggest that they use the trance preventively as well as at the first sign of any muscle tenseness, visual aura, or headache discomfort, and that the more they use the trance, the less often they will be bothered by any discomfort. It is sometimes also useful to tell children and their parents that initially the child should take whatever medication is normally used and then utilize self-hypnosis. If this combination is successful (generally relief is stronger and faster than usual) we suggest that the next time they take half as much of their normal medication and use self-hypnosis; the next time, to try one-fourth the usual amount of medication, and finally only self-hypnosis. This progression tends to yield a great deal of success, build confidence in the hypnotherapy and, increase the child's sense of control and confidence. Most children who practice self-hypnosis routinely for three or four weeks experience a significant decrease in the severity and frequency of migraine or tension headaches, gain the ability to stop a headache entirely, or markedly decrease their level of discomfort.

Further Considerations

We have attempted to describe, in some detail, how hypnotherapy can be useful in certain common pediatric medical problems, but this discussion has not by any means been exhaustive. We have also used self-hypnosis with many other chronic illnesses to (1) increase tolerance for procedures, (2) decrease specific fears (e.g., needles), (3) increase adherence to medical regimes, (e.g., medication, diet, or physical constraints), and (4) increase feelings of general well-being. Some dermatological problems such as eczema, warts, and some cases of hives are also amenable to hypnosis. Children with cerebral palsy have also been helped to decrease spasticity and increase muscular control. Many dentists have been fairly innovative in using hypnotherapy with children, and some of the children to whom we have taught self-hypnosis for other reasons have had extractions and root canals using only self-hypnosis for anesthesia. Additionally, self-hypnosis can help children relax during examinations that might be uncomfortable and/or embarrassing for them, such as pelvic or rectal exams.

In general, we believe that hypnotherapy is a useful tool in a wide range of children's physical problems, either as an adjunctive or primary means of treatment. It is important to remember, however, that any child who presents with a physical symptom should be medically evaluated and treated, if indicated, either prior to or concurrently with hypnotherapy.

SUMMARY

It is our experience that self-hypnosis is both a useful and fun technique to use with children, and we encourage professionals to use it when emotional aspects play a causative or contributory role in a child's disorder. We also encourage more and better-controlled research studies utilizing hypnotherapy with children in order to broaden its application and utilization.

REFERENCES

Agle, D.P. (1964). Psychiatric studies of patients with hemophilia and related states. *Archives of Internal Medicine, 114*, 76–82.

Ambrose, G. (1968). Hypnosis in the treatment of children. *American Journal of Clinical Hypnosis, 11*, 1–5.

Ambrose, G., & Newbold, G. (1968). *A handbook of medical hypnosis.* Baltimore: Williams & Wilkins.

American Psychiatric Association (1980). *Diagnostic and statistical manual of mental disorders* (Ed. 3). Washington, D.C.: American Psychiatric Association

Browne, W.J., Mally, M.A., & Kane, R.P. (1960). Psychosocial aspects of hemophilia: A study of twenty-eight hemophilic children and their families. *American Journal of Orthopsychiatry, 30*, 730–740.

Call, J.D. (1976). Children, parents, and hypnosis: A discussion. *International Journal of Clinical and Experimental Hypnosis, 24*, 149–155.

Cohen, H.D., Goodenough, D.R., & Witkin, H.A. (1975). The effects of stress on components of the respiratory cycle. *Psychophysiology, 12*, 377–380.

Cohen, M.W. (1975). Eneuresis. *Pediatric Clinics of North America, 22*, 545–560.

Collison, D.R. (1975). Which asthmatic patients should be treated with hypnotherapy? *Medical Journal of Australia, 1*, 107–113.

Cooper, L.M., & London, P. (1976). Children's hypnotic susceptibility, personality, and EEG patterns. *International Journal of Clinical and Experimental Hypnosis, 24*, 140–148.

Erickson, M.H. (1958). Pediatric hypnotherapy. *American Journal of Clinical Hypnosis, 1*, 25–29.

Estabrooks, G.H. (1962). *Hypnosis: Current problems.* New York: Harper & Row.

Gardner, G.G. (1974). Hypnosis with children. *International Journal of Clinical and Experimental Hypnosis, 22*, 20–38.

Gardner, G.G., & Olness, K. (1981). *Hypnosis and hypnotherapy with children.* New York: Grune & Stratton.

Hartley, R.B. (1968). Hypnosis for alleviation of pain in the treatment of burns: Case report. *Archives of Physical Medicine and Rehabilitation, 49*, 39–40.

Hilgard, E.R., & Hilgard, J.R. (1975). *Hypnosis in the relief of pain.* Los Altos, CA: William Kaufmann.

Hilgard, J.R.(1970). *Personality and hypnosis: A study of imaginative involvement.* Chicago: University of Chicago Press.

Horne, D.J. (1977). Behaviour therapy for trichotillmonania. *Behaviour Research and Therapy. 15*, 192–196.

Kahn, A.U. (1973). Present status of psychsomatic aspects of asthma. *Psychosomatics, 14*, 195–200.

Kahn, A.U., Staerk, M., & Bonk, C. (1974). Hypnotic suggestibility compared with other methods of isolating emotionally prone asthmatic children. *American Journal of Clinical Hypnosis, 17*, 50–53.

Krojanker, R.J. (1969). Human hypnosis, animal hypnotic states, and the induction of sleep in infants. *American Journal of Clinical Hypnosis, 11*, 178–179.

LaBaw, J.L., & LaBaw, W.L. (1977). Summer mountain workshops for hemophiliacs learning hypnosis. *Abstracts: Sixth World Congress of Psychiatry*, p. 258.

LaBaw, W.L. (1970). Regular use of suggestibility by pediatric bleeders. *Haemotologia,* *4,* 419–425.

LaBaw, W.L. (1973). Adjunctive trance therapy with severely burned children. *International Journal of Child Psychotherapy, 2,* 80–92.

LaBaw, W.L. (1975). Auto-hypnosis in haemophilia. *Haemotologia, 9,* 103–110.

LaBaw, W.L., Holton, C., Tewell, K., & Eccles, D. (1975). The use of self-hypnosis by children with cancer. *American Journal of Clinical Hypnosis, 17,* 233–238.

London, P. (1963). *The children's hypnotic susceptibility scale.* Palo Alto, CA: Consulting Psychologists Press.

London, P., & Masden, C.H. (1969). Role playing and hypnotic susceptibility in children. *International Journal of Clinical and Experimental Hypnosis, 17,* 37–49.

Long, T.E. (1969). Some early-life stimulus correlates of hypnotizability. *International Journal of Clinical and Experimental Hypnosis, 16,* 61–67.

Mattsson, A., & Gross, S. (1966). Adaptational and defensive behavior in young hemophiliacs and their parents. *American Journal of Psychiatry, 122,* 1349–1356.

Morgan, A., & Hilgard, J.R. (1979). Stanford hypnotic clinical scale for children. *American Journal of Clinical Hypnosis, 21,* 155–169.

Mussen, P.H., Conger, J.J., & Kagan, J. (1963). *Child development and personality* (ed. 2). New York: Harper & Row.

Nowlis, D.P. (1969). The child-rearing antecedents of hypnotic susceptibility and of naturally occurring hypnotic-like experience. *International Journal of Clinical and Experimental Hypnosis, 17,* 109–120.

Olness, K. (1981a). Imagery (self-hypnosis) as adjunct therapy in childhood cancer: Clinical experience with 25 patients. *American Journal of Pediatric Hematology/Oncology, 3,* 313–321.

Olness, K. (1981b). Hypnosis with children. *Current Problems in Pediatrics, 12,* 1–47.

Olness, K., & McDonald, J. (1981). Self-hypnosis and biofeedback in the management of juvenile migraine. *Developmental and Behavioral Pediatrics, 2,* 168–170.

Shor, R.E., & Orne, M.T. (1965). *The nature of hypnosis.* New York: Holt, Reinhart and Winston.

Spencer, R.F. (1971). Psychiatric impairment versus adjustment in hemophilia: Review and five case studies. *Psychiatry in Medicine, 2,* 1–12.

Steinhausen, H.C. (1975). A psycho-clinical investigation in adult hemophiliacs. *Journal of Psychosomatic Research, 19,* 295–302.

Udolf, R. (1981). *Handbook of hypnosis for professionals.* New York: Van NostrandReinhold.

Wakeman, R.J., & Kaplan, J.Z. (1978). An experimental study of hypnosis in painful burns. *American Journal of Clinical Hypnosis, 21,* 3–12.

11

Use of Mutual Metaphor with a Disturbed Child: A Case Study

Marie Stoner

Picture a child listening intently to a story. As that image develops in your mind, you may notice that the child is quiet, with attention focused on the story. His or her eyes may appear slightly glazed, and there is probably relaxation of the facial muscles and even the entire body. Movement is at a minimum. This child is in a natural trance state.

Storytelling can be a very potent trance induction for a child. The allusion to the child's problems and suggestions for change can transform a story into a metaphor. If this metaphor is delivered while the child is in trance, the story itself is hypnotic treatment.

Metaphoric learning depends on the psychological concept of displacement. It is often easier for a child to relate to conflicts through the distance of a story. And when suggestions for change are well embedded in the story, conscious defenses are not activated. Milton H. Erickson was a master at the art of threading a tale through conscious defenses, so that a story about a rose growing could become a metaphor for life and death. David Gordon (1978) stressed the importance of the story having a high degree of personal meaning for the patient. The story of the rose is probably most helpful to a gardener, but may even have an adverse effect on a patient highly allergic to roses. Herein lies the dilemma for most of us interested in using metaphors in hypnotherapy: how to develop a metaphor with a therapeutic meaning to the patient.

The technique illustrated in this chapter provides a model for developing a meaningful metaphor with the child in treatment. This model also draws upon Richard Gardner's Mutual Storytelling Technique. Gardner's method involves the patient and therapist trading stories and the therapist interpreting the content of the stories. The following account represents this author's attempt to utilize the receptive state of trance to suggest a healthy solution to a conflict experienced by a child. The mutuality of the metaphor allows heightened conscious and unconscious identification with the solution offered.

SARAH

Sarah was a 6-year-old first grader whose parents presented her for treatment on the recommendation of a school psychologist. In class, her behavior was reported to be withdrawn. At home, Sarah would bang her head on the table when unable to do homework assignments. She frequently cried when she arrived home from school. She also cried and was generally restless in her sleep. Psychological testing revealed an anxious child with above-average intelligence and strong perfectionistic tendencies.

Since the age of 2, Sarah had experienced physical discomfort from a combination of allergies, asthma, and colitis. These psychosomatic conditions were severe enough to have necessitated periodic hospitalizations of up to five days' duration. Her medications included cortisone and a tranquilizer for sleep disturbance.

During an initial session with Sarah's parents, the family context in which these problems had developed was explored. Sarah was the oldest of three siblings in an intact, upwardly mobile suburban family. Her father held a middle-management job which he described as "tense." Her mother was a homemaker who was hypersensitive to Sarah's distress, both physical and emotional. She would often watch out the window as Sarah played and run to her if she fell or cried. She was also spending several hours a night on homework with Sarah.

Sarah's parents did not view her medical problems as psychologically related, and it was readily apparent why this was so: Sarah's two younger siblings and her mother had various degrees of allergies and asthma, and her father was under medical treatment for an ulcer. This was a family in which the somatic expression of feelings was the normal state of affairs. However, they were concerned about their oldest child's failure to perform in first grade up to her potential and their expectations.

Treatment plans were discussed and were defined as (1) short-term individual therapy for Sarah to ameliorate her performance anxiety, and (2) consultation with her mother. As treatment progressed, this consultation with Sarah's mother revolved around the issue of increased emotional outlets within the family. Sarah's father had expressed an inability to be intimately involved in treatment due to job demands, but he did agree to be available when necessary. Both parents were cooperative with requests.

The first impression of Sarah was of a child who tried very hard to please. Her polite demeanor was punctuated by a look of concern not in keeping with her young age. She was able to acknowledge that she was "worried" in school and while doing her homework, although she did not know why she was worried or how to stop. A short explanation of therapy elicited from Sarah her cooperation in working together to get "less worry and more fun" in her life.

The primary treatment modality was a metaphor developed with Sarah over five sessions. Using information and impressions gathered from interviewing parents and child, this author formulated a treatment goal of increased awareness and expression of feelings. The metaphor was always pointed in that direction. A corollary to that goal, which was not discussed with parents or child, was the prediction that reaching this goal would have a significant impact on Sarah's psychosomatic disorders.

Each session started with general conversation with Sarah about her life. Special emphasis was placed on the ways in which she had had fun since our last appointment. After our work on the metaphor was completed, Sarah would be dismissed and the remainder of the session devoted to giving her mother an opportunity to discuss childrearing issues.

In the initial treatment session, Sarah was introduced to the trance experience through a discussion of "how we can make pictures inside our heads." Sarah, who had been described by her mother as a TV addict, was an excellent visualizer and was eager to practice describing the pictures she was able to see in her mind. For the child who finds it difficult to visualize, the concept of internal processing can be explained as "how we tell ourselves stories inside our heads." The hypnotist's geniune interest in the child's imaginative excursions is crucial and can do much to establish rapport, which is a necessary component of the trance relationship. The importance of being interested has led this author to a study of comic book characters, such as the Superheroes, rereading *Grimm's Fairy Tales*, and two viewings of "E.T.: The Extraterrestrial."

The induction of a light trance was brought about by asking Sarah to sit still and relax all the muscles in her body while she took three deep breaths. At this point, she was instructed to turn on the special TV screen in her mind. Suggestions for comfort and increasing ease with using her TV screen were given. After a discussion of that experience, cooperation was obtained for "making a movie" (or "writing a story") together.

The structure of the session in which the metaphor was developed was as follows:

    1. A light trance state would be induced by asking Sarah to close her eyes and turn on the special TV screen she had in there while she was taking three deep breaths.

    2. When Sarah showed outward signs of a relaxed state, the author would read to her the beginning of the metaphor. The story would end at a point where Sarah could make some choice regarding the direction of the metaphor.

    3. The author would ask Sarah, "What happens next?" If her response was unclear, she would be asked to go back to the TV screen and fill in the details.

    4. The following session would consist of the author reading all that had been constructed previously, plus a segment that had been added, once again ending at a point where Sarah would respond.

    5. At the end of our work on the metaphor, Sarah would be asked to close

her eyes and count from one to five as she came back from the story to the here and now.

The following story represents the combined efforts of this author and Sarah to develop a therapeutic metaphor. The metaphor drew to a natural close after five sessions, as did Sarah's treatment. Her contributions to the story are the italicized portions, written down by the author as Sarah described the picture in her mind. This picture was sometimes filled in by asking Sarah questions about what she was seeing. These details were also included in the story. Sarah's response to this method was enthusiastic. Typically, children worked with using this technique don't question its meaning. Their contributions are usually minimal, but they are able to help shape the story by their input.

Session 1

This is going to be a story about a little girl named Susie. Susie cares very much about the world and the people around her. Sometimes things people say and do make her feel hurt. But then she realizes that people don't mean to hurt her. They have their own problems and that is why they sometimes sound angry or annoyed.

Susie loves her family very much. Her mother is a beautiful lady and Susie would like to grow up to be like her someday. Susie's father is a lot of fun. He likes to make jokes, and when the whole family is laughing together Susie is very happy and relaxed.

Sometimes Susie's parents don't laugh. Sometimes they seem sad. When Susie sees this, she feels sad also. One day, Susie asked her mother what was wrong. *Her mother said that nothing was wrong.* But Susie knew that something was bothering her and she hoped that her mother was not sad about her. What her mother didn't tell Susie was that she was getting a cold. Susie thought and thought and tried to figure it out. Susie asked her daddy what was wrong with her mother. *Daddy said that she felt sick.* Susie felt a little bit better, but she still wondered. *So Susie went and watched "Caspar" on TV and* thought.

Discussion

The metaphor starts out with a general description of Susie (Sarah)'s family. Her oversensitivity to others is acknowledged and her identification with her mother is validated. Sarah's father is included in the story through the characteristic that Sarah had previously labeled as her favorite thing about him—his joking. Starting a mutual metaphor in this general way allows the child to get accustomed to the method and tests the child's ability to identify with the story.

In Sarah's case, identification with this family in the story was assured by her contribution that "nothing was wrong" with Susie's mother. Denial of negative emotions was the first line of defense in Sarah's family. When pushed to give more of an explanation of what Susie's mother wasn't telling, Sarah responded with the next line of defense: "She was getting a cold." This translation of negative emotions into somatic expression was also typical of Sarah's family and was supported by the daddy in the story: "Daddy said that she felt sick." Sarah's final contribution during the first session was to have Susie escape into television in response to the anxiety of knowing that something was wrong, but not knowing what it was.

This session fulfills the first requirement of a therapeutic metaphor, which is to map out the unhealthy pattern.

Session 2

Inside her head Susie started to imagine a story. And the story went like this:

Once upon a time in a kingdom far from here and closer to there, there was a city of people with thin skins. Now you may wonder what people with thin skins look like. Well, let me tell you, they look very much like you or like me. They had eyes with which they could see what was going on around them, and very good ears with which to hear all that was said. The only way in which they were different is that the distance between their insides and their outsides was smaller than in people we know.

Their city was bright and warm and they were very happy, laughing and playing all day long. You can imagine them singing and running and talking to each other in happy voices. Because their city was so warm and bright, their thin skins were never a problem, and Susie's story would have been happy if it had ended here.

But one morning the thin skinned people woke up, stretched their thin-skinned bodies, and all of a sudden started shivering. The bravest among them rushed outdoors and there they saw *it was raining outside. There were clouds in the sky. They were not used to it raining. The kids felt sad because they couldn't go out to play. They cried and cried until their thin skins got rough and itched.* Then they were really miserable because they were crying and scratching. *They didn't know what to do.*

Discussion

This author's choice to transfer the story to a fantasy setting was based on a truth known to all lovers of children's literature: that a setting "far from here" allows the child to think in new ways. The thin-skinned people are a representation of Sarah's family in their physical and emotional sensitivity to stress. Once again, Sarah is asked to contribute the part of the story that explains what has upset these thin-skinned people (just as she was asked in the first session to explain what was bothering Susie's mother). Once again, Sarah externalized her explanation of what had upset these people: "It was raining outside." Their crying caused their thin skins to get rough and itch (a clear psychosomatic reference). As in the first session, we have the unhealthy pattern of uncomfortable emotions becoming translated into physical discomfort.

Session 3

Among the thin-skinned people was one small person with long legs and long hair whose name was Chantell. Chantell was itching and scratching just like the rest of the thin-skinned people, but she decided that she wanted to be happy. She wanted to help herself and her friends, but she didn't know exactly how.

Chantell remembered that once in a dream she had been told about a magic tree in the middle of the city park. She decided to visit the tree and see what happened. So she went scratching and crying to the magic tree. By the time she got there, she was so tired that she sat under the tree and fell asleep.

Suddenly she saw, or maybe she dreamt that she saw, a lovely fairy floating down from the top branch of the tree. The fairy landed right by her feet and sat down beside her smiling a beautiful smile. She said, "Dear Chantell, you really are so brave to come out in all this rain to find me. What can I do for you?"

Chantell said, "Oh, things are so terrible! My friends and I are all scratching and crying. Can you help us?"

The fairy looked carefully to all sides, twirled around three times and said, "Chantell, I can see that you are unhappy. You would like to have this city the way that it used to be, always sunny and warm. But my magic powers cannot stop the rain. Things can never be the way that they used to be. At times it will rain, and at times the sun will come out. But Dear Chantell, I would like to help you and your friends stop itching and crying and I will do anything within my powers to help. I will grant you three magic wishes to help you feel better. What would your wishes be?"

Chantell sat and thought. She felt sad that the rain had come into the kingdom of thin-skinned people, but she knew that the fairy couldn't stop the rain. She thought carefully, then she gave her wishes, which were:

1. *Help me and my friends stop itching.*
2. *Help me and my friends stop crying.*
3. *And I would like a horse.*

Discussion

What turns a child's story into a therapeutic metaphor is the suggestion of a healthy resolution to conflict. Instead of withdrawing as Susie or Sarah did, Chantell was able to ask for help. There are many guises for a helpful figure. a 6-year-old girl such as Sarah certainly would listen to a lovely fairy, but a 10-year-old boy might need to be introduced to a kung fu master.

The fairy imparts a significant message to Chantell that sets a framework for change, and that is the insistence that "things can never be the way they used to be." Sarah's psychosomatic symptoms started shortly after the birth of her sister, and it can be assumed that part of her conflict had to do with her desire to return to a time before the pressures of school and before her brother and sister joined the family.

Session 4

The fairy said, "I will grant your wishes. Come back to this magic tree tomorrow when the shadows of evening are just starting. But, in the meantime, I have a very important job for you to do." The fairy went on to say, "I have lived in this magic tree for many years. And I have watched the thin-skinned people come and go around me. I love your people, Chantell. But one thing has bothered me and I want you to help me with it.

Because the thin-skinned people have so little space between their insides and their outsides, they are very afraid to let their feelings get loose. I've noticed that your people .walk around with all their feelings inside their bodies. This makes me sad because feelings are very special to me. They come in so many different shapes and colors. There's the red of anger, the peaceful blue of calm, and the green of jealousy. Each feeling is good and proper in its own way. Feelings are what make people able to see me and believe in me. Because you knew that you were unhappy and were able to tell me that you were unhappy, you were able to see me. The job I want you to do during the next day is to help the rest of the thin-skinned people have feelings. Then many more people will be able to see me and I will have lots of friends. If you can help me with my problem, then I will gladly grant you the three wishes."

Chantell left the park, happy that she was going to get her three wishes, but puzzled as to how she was going to help the thin-skinned people let their feelings out. Being a brave girl, she decided to give it a try. She gathered together all the thin-skinned people in the city. And what a noise it was with all of them in one place! Crying and wailing and scratching! Finally she had to stand on top of a milk crate so that she could be heard over all the noise. And this is what she said to them: "*Thin-skinned people, try not to worry.*"

One of the adults standing there said, "Not worry! Why, There are so many things to worry about. Why should I stop worrying?"

Chantell told him, "*If you try not to worry, then your feelings will come out. And if your feelings come out, I will get my wishes and we will all stop scratching and crying.*"

Naturally, it took quite a bit of convincing for all of the people to agree with Chantell. Finally they said they would try to let their feelings out. One little boy looked at Chantell and said, "I don't know how not to worry. Can you tell me how?"

Chantell said, "Of course. *You just try not to think of worrying about things. Get busy when you start to worry. Have fun. And if you're still worried, take a glass of water.*

Discussion

At this point in the metaphor, the therapeutic change is introduced. The fairy suggests to Chantell that the expression of feelings will make her wishes come true. But it is left to Chantell (Sarah) to figure out a way for the thin-skinned people to let their feelings out. Sarah's important contribution during this session is the recognition that "worry" (anxiety) is blocking the expression of feeling. In order to obtain specific recommendations for dealing with anxiety, Sarah was urged to keep looking at the picture on her TV screen as the adult and the boy questioned her. It is Sarah's insight that this anxiety can be dissipated by staying busy and having fun.

Session 5

The thin-skinned people practiced all of the next day and were still trying not to worry when Chantell made her trip to the magic tree. The fairy was waiting for her at the base of the tree and she had a big smile on her face. She said, "Chantell, you did a very good job. The thin-skinned people are showing their feelings like they never have before and it makes me very happy! I'm sure that I'll have many friends now."

Chantell was excited because she knew that she would get her wishes. The fairy knew what Chantell was thinking. She said, "Chantell, your first two wishes have already been granted. You wanted the itching and crying to stop. What you don't know is that by teaching the thin-skinned people how to stop worrying and start showing their feelings, you have made your wishes come true."

Chantell didn't really understand. She did remember that she herself hadn't itched or cried since she had told the fairy about her own feelings the day before. And she was happy and proud that she had been the one to teach the thin-skinned people this important thing.

The fairy continued, "And since you have done such a good job and have helped your people, I have a gift for you." From behind a bush, she brought a beautiful brown and white spotted pony. Chantell jumped on the pony's back and happily waved goodbye to the fairy as she rode away. As she rode through the town, she discovered that what the fairy had said was true. Nobody was scratching and crying. All the thin-skinned people were showing their feelings, just as Chantell had asked them to. Happy people, sad people . . . but none were scratching.

Chantell was very, very happy as she rode on. And all of a sudden, she felt a new feeling. And that was *liking herself*. And that's the best feeling of all.

Discussion

The story ends happily, with wishes coming true and a new pattern established. Chantell and Sarah don't really understand how the expression of feelings led to the symptoms of scratching and crying disappearing. If a metaphor is well designed, conscious understanding is not necessary and may even interfere with the child's readiness to accept the changes suggested in the story. Sarah was never asked to make conscious connections between Chantell and herself. She was simply asked to help make a movie.

The buildup of the metaphor over the five sessions meant that more and more of Sarah's time in each session was devoted to hearing the story read one more time and adding on a new segment. The sixth session, which was a final session, consisted of the telling of the entire metaphor without interruption while Sarah was in a light trance. She was then presented with a copy of the story to take home, to which she responded with a great deal of pride.

CONCLUSION

The six treatment sessions occurred over a period of 11 weeks. One month after we started the story, the mother mentioned that Sarah's allergy doctor had reduced her medication. The parents did not connect this change with any shifts in Sarah's behavior. On further inquiry in a subsequent session, it was reported that not only were her allergic episodes less frequent and less severe, but she had had no asthma or colitis attacks and her sleep was peaceful. By the end of our work on the story, Sarah was off all medication.

Feedback from the classroom started improving at about the same rate. Sarah's grades during the report period following referral went from Bs to some Bs and some As. Her teacher reported increased classroom participation and less observable anxiety. In a parent-teacher conference, the teacher shared an unusual piece of behavior. During a math test, Sarah had raised her hand to tell the teacher that she was worried and would like to get a drink of water. Chantell's recommendations had been carried into the classroom.

There have been two follow-up conversations with Sarah's mother. One month after treatment ended, Sarah was still off all medication and had completed first grade quite successfully. An inquiry in the early months of second grade revealed that Sarah had maintained her improvement. She had experienced some allergic reactions over the summer, but her other physical problems had not resurfaced, and she was happily adjusted in school.

The use of a mutual metaphor is applicable to a variety of clinical situations. A child faced with difficult or painful medical procedures can rehearse coping strategies through the eyes of a child in a story who may be facing a dragon of a different sort. The child will respond to the threat in the story in an idiosyncratic fashion, allowing the clinician to hear what will work to lower stress in the way that asking for a drink of water helped Sarah to cope with her test anxiety.

On occasion, a child will ask what the story means, or whether the story is about them. These questions should be responded to directly. The child may be satisfied with an explanation that working on the story will help with a problem. On the other hand these inquiries may be a signal that the child is uncomfortable with the ambiguity of the storytelling situation and would prefer a more direct counseling or hypnotic strategy.

Giving the child the choice of sharing the story with his or her family raises another level of intervention as parents struggle to make sense of this strange form of therapy. Sarah's parents obviously got the message of the metaphor since her mother called several months after termination to inquire about stress management courses to help her husband's ulcer. A child's desire to keep the story private should be respected. There is probably a good reason for that choice.

Most preadolescent children approached with the idea of a joint storytelling (movie-making) therapy have been receptive. It is important to have the child's conscious cooperation and vital that the child's input into the story be treated with respect. For it is the client's view of the world which must be brought to life in the metaphor, so that alternative solutions can be found to the problems of that world.

REFERENCES

Gardner, R.A. (1971). *Therapeutic communication with children.* New York: Johnson Aronson.

Gordon, D. (1978). *Therapeutic metaphors: Helping others through the looking glass.* Cupertino, CA: Meta Publications.

PART IV

Other Clinical Applications

12

Hypnosis for Weight Loss and Smoking Cessation

Eileen O'Connell

Through most of this century, health care in the United States has been primarily focused on diagnosis and treatment of illness. The recipient of the health care service was identified as the passive "patient." Interest in prevention was low, partly because the general concensus predicted medical breakthroughs that would soon cure many diseases. Because prevention of disease was not a primary focus of health care, smoking cessation and treatment of obesity problems were generally neglected. Patients were often advised to quit smoking, but no effective aid was available to assist the patient in this process, and failure rates were high. More attention was focused on the problem of weight control. However, the goal in weight control was generally oriented to cosmetic change rather than promotion of health. The primary modes of treatment were drugs such as amphetamines, or even surgical interventions. Thus, the effects of many weight control programs were physically detrimental to the patient, and provided no lasting weight loss or change in eating habits.

In recent years, attention has begun to be directed on primary prevention as a central aspect of health care service. Health maintenance and prevention of illness have become an increasing focus of professional practice. The health care recipient is now being identified as a client rather than a patient, and as someone who should have an active role in his/her own health care. Attention to prevention has been reflected in a return to interest in habit control, particularly in the areas of smoking and obesity. Smoking and obesity have longterm health implications. In addition to impairing daily activity and impeding organ function, there is increasing evidence that these habits interact with other environmental factors to promote disease and slow recovery. There is no area of practice where nursing can have a more important role in disease prevention than by helping clients who have smoking or overeating habits.

In this chapter we will discuss the major issues that encompass the problems of smoking and overeating. We will outline the steps that must be taken to set up an effective hypnosis intervention. These steps will include evaluation of the client and the habit, planning an intervention, and follow-up. Examples of specific hypnotic suggestions will be used to illustrate.

UNDERSTANDING THE PROBLEM

The problems of overeating or smoking are generally considered to be habitual difficulties. Before planning an intervention in these problem areas the therapist must first understand the nature and meaning of the term *habit*, and be familiar with the specific problems associated with smoking and overeating.

What is a Habit?

A habit is defined as an acquired mode of behavior that has become nearly or completely involuntary. In other words, it is not genetically programmed or instinctual, but learned. A habit behavior is an ongoing part of life, and usually proceeds without conscious consideration as part of a routine.

Habits can be useful or adaptive because they decrease the amount of decision making that must be done on a a daily bais. Always taking the same route to work makes one less decision necessary in the day. Always locking the door at night is a habit that most people do not even need to consider. A well-run life is composed of literally hundreds of different habits that serve to promote efficiency and minimize stress. Many times the origin of the behavior is so deeply rooted that we do not understand its meaning, but meaning does exist, often deeply lodged in the unconscious.

In planning any habit control intervention there are three components of a habit that must be addressed. These are (1) conditioned response, (2) emotional association/psychological motives, and (3) physical dependence.

Conditioned Response

Basic to the understanding of the conditioned response is the concept of the reflex arc. A reflex is an automatic response to a stimulus. The reflex response is part of the nervous system and does not require conscious thought or effort. One basic or simple reflex is the knee jerk response. When the knee is tapped, the sensory nerve sends a message to the spinal cord. In the spinal cord, the impulse is relayed to a motor nerve and back to the leg, causing the muscle to contract. This is called a simple reflex arc. It involves only two nerves and one synapse. A simple reflex does not require upper central nervous system involvement. By the time the brain receives the signal of sensation of the knee tap, the motor response, i.e. the knee jerk, has already occurred.

A similar type of reflex is the conditioned response. A conditioned response is acquired through repeated action. It is a learned response. When a behavior or action is repeated, the nervous system learns to react automatically and a new reflex is built into the nervous system. The conditioned reflex response was first documented by Pavlov in his frequently cited experiments with dogs. Pavlov delineated three phases of learning. In the first phase a perception of food was noted to lead to an increase in salivary gland activity. Pavlov then intervened by adding the sound of a bell to the perception of food. After this phase the sound of the bell alone, even when not accompanied by food, would trigger the dog's salivary gland secretion. This is a conditioned reflex.

From this series of experiments evolved the theory of classical conditioning, which states that a stimulus will serve to set off an automatically conditioned response. In the case of smokers and overeaters, the habit behavior may have, for example, initially been used as an outlet for tension during a stressful period. It was perceived as a response to stress that would allay anxiety or increase coping ability. Just as Pavlov's dogs salivate with the bell, so does the smoker or overeater respond to environmental stimuli by craving a cigarette or food. The stimulus for the craving may be a routine event such as a coffee break, or it may be a feeling such as anxiety.

In planning treatment intervention, hypnosis is aimed at creating increased awareness of the specific conditioned behavior, and then at extinction of the learned response, followed by suggestions that will serve to integrate new, healthier responses. Direct suggestion can also be used to block the impact of environmental triggers of the conditioned behavior.

Emotional Associations/Psychological Motives

In human beings the conditioned reflex (habit) is often tied to an emotional effect that has become associated with the habit. This emotional effect is usually a sense of pleasure, relaxation, or enjoyment. Pleasurable feelings create a strong reinforcement for the habit behavior. For example, many nurses begin smoking during their nursing education. At that time the behavior was a response to stress and anxiety. The act of smoking became associated to relaxation, taking a break, sitting down, momentarily experiencing some relief from emotional pressure. Over time this association (stress → smoking → relaxation) became generalized, and any stressful situation became a trigger for smoking. The emotional associations of the habit increase the difficulty of change, because the client is fighting not only the conditioned reflex behavior but is also giving up a structure that may have been a primary source of gratification or relief from anxiety. For this reason, the client will often experience an increase in anxiety or a feeling of deprivation until new, more constructive conditioned responses are developed.

Hypnosis is used to create awareness of the ways in which the client has been emotionally dependent on the behavior. A new emotional association—receiving genuine satisfaction from increased control over the habit behavior—

will be created. In addition, hypnosis is a powerful tool that can help the client counter the attempts of advertisers to create emotional dependence on their products. Self-suggestion and visual imagery can be taught to the client to help decondition and dissociate them from the advertiser's messages. Hypnosis can strengthen resistance to the triggers that advertisers set up in order to stimulate cravings for food or cigarettes. In this way we teach our clients to avoid becoming dupes of the habit salespeople.

Physical Dependence

The third aspect of a habit that must be considered is the aspect of physical dependence. Removing substances and chemicals to which the body has become accustomed can create discomfort until the body has a chance to readjust.

Hypnosis can be used to help the client reinterpret the sensations of physical distress. This use of hypnosis is similar to the way hypnosis is used in pain management. Sensations of discomfort will be more tolerable if the client feels highly motivated, and feels that the discomfort is a sign of healing and growth toward a goal.

The Smoking Habit

The U.S. Department of Health and Human Services has called smoking "the most widespread example of drug dependency in our country." The Surgeon General has cited smoking as the most important single cause of cancer mortality in the United States. In addition, it appears that the toxins in cigarettes may interact with other environmental toxins. This interaction or cocarcinogenic effect increases toxicity far beyond the effect of either chemical alone. There is probably no other area of health maintenance where the effect of nursing intervention can be so important.

As previously discussed, any intervention with a smoker must address the three components of habit: conditioned response, emotional associations, and physical dependence. Let us now examine the habit of smoking in regard to these factors.

Conditioned Response to Smoking

People who smoke as a response to conditioning can be considered routine smokers. Clients who are routine smokers will describe themselves as smoking automatically, often unaware that they have lit a cigarette. They may frequently light a cigarette without realizing that they have another one still burning in an ashtray.

They may always smoke while driving, or always smoke while drinking coffee or alcohol. Questioning the clients about rituals or times when they smoke will often identify the routine aspects of their smoking habit. Hypnosis will create increased awareness of routine as a trigger. Direct suggestion can then be used to create consciousness of the behavior and motivation to find a more constructive outlet. Example "When driving you will be aware of how good it feels to be a nonsmoker."

Emotional Aspects of Smoking

One of the effects of nicotine on the body is muscle relaxation. This creates a mild sense of well-being. The immediate benefit of smoking to a tense, anxious client can easily be seen. The effect is not usually consciously perceived by the smoker, They just try smoking, experience relief of tension, and become conditioned to smoking when anxious.

The tobacco industry has focused its attention on this emotional association between relaxation and smoking and uses powerful suggestive techniques in its advertising campaigns. Virtually all cigarette advertising is geared toward showing a situation in which relaxation or pleasure is occurring. This may be suggested directly (a couple is seen sitting by a waterfall) or it may be indirectly suggested (a man has just scaled a mountain and is now relaxing from the challenge by smoking a cigarette). The image creates an association between a cigarette and feelings of well-being, happiness, and accomplishment. We would all like to be able to purchase these emotions, and advertisers imply that we can do so by creating a happy image and then introducing a cigarette.

Some smokers have a relatively mild emotional association to cigarettes. This type of smoker can be considered a "social smoker." These people smoke occasionally and can generally quit with little difficulty. Their dependence on cigarettes may be a response to anxiety or stress. They feel a pleasurable relaxation from smoking, will often describe themselves as having a strong desire to smoke at social gatherings, and may describe the ritual of handling cigarettes as enjoyable. Their ability to quit easily tends to allow them to continue to rationalize their smoking as something they can stop at any time. The hypnotic intervention in this instance should be aimed at creating a new structure for these pleasurable sensations and decreasing the pleasure derived from the ritual of smoking. Example: "You will feel proud to be a nonsmoker, relaxed and happy about your increasing motivation to remain a nonsmoker."

Physical Dependency

Until recently, smoking was felt to create psychological dependence or habituation, but no actual physical dependence or addiction. Recent studies have indicated that of the more than 1000 different chemical compounds present in cigarettes, at least one of them, nicotine, is physically addicting. The craving for a cigarette is a physical response to receptors that have developed a bonding effect with nicotine, and these receptors signal the need for replenishing the nicotine supply. This may account for the periodic cravings that can occur even after long periods of non-smoking. It may also account for the frequently expressed desire of quitters to "sniff the air" near a smoker. The dynamics of the interaction between nicotine and neuroreceptors is not yet fully understood.

This physical need creates a type of smoker who must be characterized as an addict. These clients can be distinguished by their regular craving for a cigarette and their inability to take their mind off of the fact that they are not smoking. When strongly addicted, the smoker may wake up at night to have a cigarette, smoke upon arising in the morning, or leave a movie to have a cigarette.

As with other addictions, it is speculated that different degrees of susceptibility to nicotine addiction occur in different people. Withdrawal experience in smokers varies widely with individual physiology. Symptoms of withdrawal can include cravings, anxiety, irritability, cramps, disorientation, fatigue, or depression. In rare cases, symptoms can be of such severity that withdrawal will have to proceed under medical supervision. Complete cessation has been demonstrated to be the only effective intervention in treating substance abuse. Alcohol or drug abusers must abstain from any use, since moderating intake has not proven to be successful. Smoking is similar to other forms of substance abuse in this regard. The presence of small amounts of nicotine in the body will stimulate the neuroreceptors to call for more, this will cause, in effect, a return to withdrawal symptoms. For this reason the only effective way to quit smoking is through complete cessation. Where there is physical dependence on nicotine, hypnosis will be used to strengthen and enhance motivation (which will increase the client's ability to tolerate uncomfortable side effects of cessation) and to help the client reinterpret the discomfort of nicotine withdrawal.

The Overeating Problem

We live in a society that values boyishly slim figures for men and women: body fat is considered unattractive and unsightly. This image prevails even though there is evidence that some amount of body fat may contribute to health and longevity, and even though many people live active healthy lives with body weights that our current fashion considers overweight. People who are overweight are often viewed with disdain, and are seen having little self-regard or as simply lazy. The victims of these prejudices are acutely aware of the ways in which society discriminates against them. Affected by these attitudes, they suffer from diminished self-esteem. In addition to psychological and social difficulties, obese individuals are at risk of emotional or physical illness. Many of the health consequences of poor diet are longterm. It has been difficult to prove a definite correlation between diet and disease; conclusive links have been established between obesity and diabetes, hypertension, and heart disease.

Stunkard (1983) has identified three clinical issues that arise in treating a weight loss client: dropping out of treatment, emotional disturbances during dieting, and regaining weight. Because of the long term commitment that weight loss involves, it is crucial that a weight loss program address the three aspects of a habit.

Conditioned Response

Eating patterns are complex conditioned behaviors, set very early in life. Many of the conditioned responses to food are set in place before we are old enough to be aware of acquiring them. They are powerful parts of our daily routine. We establish a pattern of eating at certain times of the day, this becomes conditioned, and many people will experience hunger at their regular mealtime even though they have eaten only a short time before. Hypnosis will be used to create awareness of the conditioned behavior as it occurs, and allow the weight loss client to consider alternative behaviors.

Emotional Association

Conditioned responses that have been part of behavior for much of life will have strong emotional associations. Clients frequently feel anxious or depressed during the course of weight loss. One causative factor for these feelings may be the disruption of the conditioned response. Food is strongly associated with feelings: we celebrate with food, and we eat when depressed or anxious.

Physical Dependence

Many people who are overweight are heavy users of sugar. They experience cravings and depression when giving up sugar, much the way that smokers experience cravings and emotional difficulties when giving up nicotine. Some are accustomed to drinking large amounts of cola-type soft drinks; these, in addition to being heavily sugared, often contain caffeine—again precipitating withdrawal discomfort.

One of the central problems with the physical dependence on eating is that complete cessation is not possible. The client cannot stop eating altogether, but must learn moderation.

Because of the complex psychological and physiological interactions, it is important that a weight-loss intervention program satisfy certain basic needs, including (1) structure, (2) ego development, (3) supportive relationship with the therapist, and (4) peer and environmental supports.

Structured Program

In working with destructive eating habits, we are generally removing a behavior that was learned early in life. Part of what makes change so difficult in these cases is the many subtle ways in which eating behaviors have attached themselves to the client's basic life structure. In addition, people associate certain foods with feelings of comfort or pleasure. This emotional association results in a genuine sense of deprivation, loss, or anxiety when change is attempted.

For these reasons it is important that hypnosis be used as one tool in an eclectic, comprehensive weight-loss program. The intervention should include identification of the roots of the overeating problem, agreement on a reasonable time frame for weight loss, motivational support, and dietary counseling. Attention should be given to the need for longterm commitment, because this is one of the primary difficulties experienced by most weight-loss clients. Hypnotic suggestions should be aimed toward helping the client achieve a feeling of challenge. Many overweight people feel overwhelmed and discouraged by the prospect of spending an extended period of time acquiring new eating habits. By suggesting that weight loss is a process, the hypnotic integration of new ideas and patterns can be achieved over time.

The use of a cassette tape for reinforcement can provide a valuable ongoing structure to the client. The tape should include a standard induction with suggestions regarding motivation, attitude, feelings of control over food, and adherence to the diet program. It should be a summary of the issues defined in the individual session. Use of a cassette tape will be discussed further in the section on reinforcement.

Many clients report good results from keeping a food journal, which is a diary of daily food intake and calorie total. This structure provides immediate positive reinforcement for successful days and is often a source of information as clients begin to identify situations or times of day when they consume an excess of calories.

Ego Development

It is difficult to determine whether the poor self-image associated with being overweight is a cause of obseity or a result of societal attitudes about weight. There is certainly, however, a direct correlation between the desire to lose weight and poor self-image. Any weight-loss intervention should be based on the assumption that there is a poor self-image; therefore, a number of basic ego needs can be assumed to exist. Ego-development suggestions can be aimed at pride in new body appearance, the ability to maintain commitment, and the ability to change. Depression and anxiety are often commonly encountered in the course of a weight-loss program. These feelings probably have physiological as well as psychological roots (Stunkard, 1983). Hypnosis should be directed at strengthening the client's ability to comfortably maintain the required diet and to positively redirecting the normal anxiety that will occur.

Need for a Positive Relationship with the Therapist

In treating weight-loss clients, it is important for the therapist to be aware of his or her own feelings or prejudices about obesity. It is not at all unusual for us to unconsciously subscribe to the opinion that people who are overweight are weak-willed, lazy, or indifferent. This is a common attitude, even among nurses who have struggled with a weight problem themselves. These attitudes will be transmitted to the client and will disrupt the treatment relationship. Feelings of irritation or frustration on the part of the therapist about the client's rate of weight loss is often an indication that such an attitude is present. The client will respond most positively to a therapeutic relationship that is nonjudgmental and supportive without promoting unnecessary dependence.

Because the hypnotist is an authority figure, it is also common for transference to occur. For example, the client may project onto the therapist feelings of nonsupport or criticism, which indicate the client's own internal state. These feelings tend to emerge early in the treatment relationship. The possibility of transference should be considered if the client seems hostile, unduly challenging, or resistant. This phenomenon is one of the reasons that hypnosis for weight loss is particularly effective in groups. The group setting serves to diffuse the intensity of transference and provides reality testing about whether the problem is based in the client's attitude or the therapist's prejudices.

The Need for Peer and Environmental Support

Many people who are trying to lose weight spend a lot of time comparing notes with other dieters, gauging their "success," and juggling calories. The client may benefit from having other people available who are engaged in the same change process. Peer support can be a powerful motivator and is particularly important for those who do not receive support from family or friends.

TREATMENT

Treatment of a smoking or weight problem should be based upon an understanding of the nature of these habits. The use of hypnosis should be part of a holistic approach that moves through a series of planned phases: assessment, formulating a treatment plan, and reinforcement and follow-up.

Assessment Phase

The goal of assessment is to obtain a full understanding of the nature of the habit, its role in the client's life, and the client's capacity for change. The first step is to determine the appropriateness of treating the habit. Smoking and overeating may be symptoms of underlying problems. In these cases, the modification of the habit can have unforseen side effects because the client may not be emotionally ready to withstand the stress created by change. For this reason, a screening similar to a standard psychiatric interview should be considered. The client should be evaluated for symptoms of underlying depression, psychotic thought processes, use of psychotropic medications, history of psychological difficulties, or suicidal ideation. Evidence of any of the above signals the need for thorough exploration of the client's reason for seeking habit change. Once the client has been deemed a suitable candidate for a habit-control intervention, the process of determining the client's capacity for change can begin.

Capacity for change is not a fixed, predetermined state, but is rather a result of many factors. These factors include innate hypnotizability, motivation, strength of the habit, and a structure for change that meets individual personality needs. In the course of the assessment the therapist will evaluate all of these factors. Spiegel and Spiegel (1978) suggested that cases be seen as puzzles; in the assessment phase the therapist must determine which are the most important pieces.

Hypnotizability

Hypnotizability has proven, over the course of many years and numerous research projects, to be extremely difficult to predict. There have been innumerable attempts to relate hypnotic ability to specific single traits such as gender, eye color, or intelligence. These attempts have been largely fruitless. The most promising correlation for trance capacity seems to be that hypnotizability is related to a basic general personality style. There appear to be certain styles of thinking that are associated with high hypnotic ability. Generally speaking, people who fall into the high trance capacity tend to be characterized as trusting, having a good memory, and the capacity for intense and focused concentration. They are people who are flexible when considering new ideas and new events. People with low hypnotizability tend to be highly cognitive, organized, critical, and place a great deal of emphasis on reason and understanding (see also Chapter 2).

Innate hypnotizability is an important and valuable asset for the client in habit control. However, there are a number of other factors that can increase or decrease the capacity of the client to use hypnosis as a tool in smoking cessation or weight control.

Motivation

In addition to innate hypnotizability, motivation is a crucial factor in the successful use of hypnosis as a tool in weight loss or smoking control. An understanding of the client's motivation is particularly important when the therapist suspects that the client is a marginal or a poor subject in terms of innate hypnotizability. Some clients who appear to be difficult subjects to hypnotize will have success because their motivation is high. The therapist should attempt to gain an understanding of the internal desire and motivation to change the habit.

In modifying a smoking or overeating habit the client will have to be motivated to follow the treatment program over an extended period to time. This allows the necessary conditioning to take place. People who come seeking magical cures or desire rapid change without effort will generally become disappointed when they experience difficulty that they abandon treatment. If the client is attempting to stop smoking or lose weight because of peer or family pressure (external motivators) rather than a genuine desire to change, then internal motivation is not high. In this case, the use of hypnosis is not likely to be able to provide sufficient impact on the subject. On the other hand, if internal motivation is high then the use of hypnosis will be greatly enhanced, even in subjects who would be considered poor in terms of innate ability. When internal motivation is high, then external motivating factors such as family or peer supports can greatly promote success.

Direct suggestion can be very useful to enhance motivation. Typical suggestions should directly state the client's own desire to change and commitment to following the prescribed regimen. (*Example*: "You will be motivated to be a nonsmoker, because this is a decision that *you* have made, because this is something that *you* choose").

Drive to Continue the Habit

In addition to motivation the therapist should also examine the drive to continue the habit. How much genuine pleasure is derived from the behavior? Is the physical experience completely satisfying, or are there aspects that are distasteful to the client? Determining which aspects of the habit are negatively perceived will aid the therapist in directing suggestion.

One important aspect of drive is secondary gain. Secondary gain refers to the unconscious reward or benefit that is derived from the habit. For example, a smoker may enjoy the attention shown by family members who are concerned about his or her health. Expressions of concern paid to physical side effects of the behavior (such as smoker's cough) are common examples of secondary gain. A realistic appraisal of the emotional losses that will be incurred by the habit change will increase the therapist's ability to formulate an effective hypnosis intervention.(*Example*: "You will experience feelings of pride, and others notice your change.")

Feelings

It will be common to find that thoughts and feelings about the habit are in direct conflict. The client may, for example, *know* that quitting smoking would be in his or her own best interest. However, the client may *feel* that smoking is enjoyable and relaxing. Creating congruence between thinking and feelings will be an important aspect of the suggestion process. (*Example*: "You will begin to feel differently when you see someone smoking now. You will not envy them, you'll feel sorry for them because you know that they are destroying their body with their dependence on this poison. You will be proud that you no longer need to smoke." *or* "As you begin to change your eating habits you will be proud of your new found ability to desire healthy foods.").

Etiology and History of the Habit

The therapist should determine the circumstances under which the habit began. Were there any life stressors at the time of the onset of the behavior? If so, what purpose did the habit initially serve? Determining the circumstances of onset is useful because direct and indirect suggestion can be geared to restructuring the learned response. In some subjects, a hypnotic regression to the initial experience will often provide information about precipitating events. During the hypnotic regression many smokers will identify adolescence as the time of onset and will cite peer pressure as the most important trigger to the initial desire to smoke. This information can then be integrated as a direct suggestion during the hypnotic induction. (*Example*: "You have outgrown your need to smoke to be part of a group. You are confident and assured of your ability to be smoke-free in any social situation.")

In obtaining a history of the habit, the therapist should examine the course the habit has taken in the client's life. This course includes periods of increased or decreased habit behavior, as for example, periods of weight loss or gain, and the time that weight loss was maintained. The therapist should attempt to determine the precipitating cause of relapse, which is often a major stressful life event. The client will often not associate the stressful event with the relapse. In these cases, the therapist should help the client to understand this causal relationship, as stressful life events are sure to occur in the future. Posthypnotic suggestions can be particularly useful here to set up an automatic relaxation response when the client is stressed. (*Example*: "When you are stressed, or when you experience a craving, you will rub your thumb and forefinger together. This will relax you and you will find that the craving will fade.")

Historical data should also include information about attempts to change. If the client has tried many different treatment approaches before seeking a hypnosis intervention and describes each method as having failed them, then this client may be someone who is seeking a pain-free approach to change. Clients who are angry and easily disappointed in previous attempts to change have a high likelihood of repeating this pattern unless some action is taken to help them gain a genuine commitment. The therapist should help the client to interpret this past behavior and understand the need for an active commitment to the change process.

Triggers for the Habit

A trigger is an internal or external event that creates the desire to smoke; it sets off the unconscious conditioned response. For a smoker, the trigger may be driving, drinking coffee, or feeling social pressures. For a weight-control client, the trigger may be boredom or anxiety, or it may be taking a coffee break, which "must" include a doughnut.

Suggestions should be aimed at these specific triggers, and the hypnosis program should include a redirection of the conditioned response to other behaviors. Sometimes the client may be able to avoid some trigger situations. Encouraging a client who is quitting smoking to avoid coffee and alcohol may be helpful, because these are two common triggers. A weight-loss client may need to initially avoid situations (e.g., coffee breaks) in which he or she is prone to eating foods that are not part of the diet. The client may need to avoid the trigger event with the behavior. When the trigger situation is reintroduced, a reprogrammed behavior will be introduced at the same time, such as an internal attitude of "I never have doughnuts, only coffee, at my coffee break."

Trigger situations cannot be avoided forever, and many, such as driving or eating dinner, cannot be avoided at all. In these cases the use of strong direct suggestion will be useful in helping the client introduce new learned responses. (*Example*: "You will find that when you are driving you will experience pleasure in knowing that you are now a nonsmoker." *or* "During a coffee break you will avoid snacks and fattening foods. You will not notice them. You will forget that they are available. If you are offered an unhealthy food, you will refuse. This will immediately make you feel proud of your new abilities to have your mind in control of your body.")

Treatment Phase

Once the assessment process is complete the therapist has the information to design a treatment plan that is comprehensive, in-depth and personalized.

Treatment should be directed at both conscious and unconscious levels of the mind. Consciously, discussion, support and information sharing can be used as interventions. Building unconscious motivation through subtle suggestion enhances a positive outcome. Hypnosis then is directed toward change on both the conscious and unconscious level.

In developing a treatment plan, a number of considerations are important. They include (1) the nature of the therapist–client relationship; (2) types of hypnotic suggestions; (3) an appropriate timeline for reaching the goal or number of sessions planned; and (4) other types of interventions that will be used.

Therapist–Client Relationship

Many people approach the use of hypnosis with uncertainty and suspicion. The view of a hypnotist as someone who may try to control, influence, or otherwise affect the client is still a common fear for most people who have never experienced hypnosis. The most effective way to counter this fear is by the development of a collegial relationship in which the client feels that he or she has an active part in determining the course of treatment. This relationship can be considered a therapeutic alliance, with the therapist and the client working together to achieve their goal.

There is evidence that clients who are poor or marginal subjects will benefit from explanation of the treatment plan and indeed may want a great deal of input into specific suggestions. For these clients or for those who are markedly anxious, it is not unreasonable for the therapist to spend most or all of an initial session answering questions and defining treatment interventions. On the other hand, clients who can quickly develop trusting relationships will generally desire much less input into specific aspects of the treatment plan and will often be confused if too much is spent in detailing specifics.

Types of Hypnotic Suggestions*

Evidence exists that highly authoritarian suggestions can bring about client resistance. Boris Sidis (1898) found that "this approach brought out in many clients a desire to resist, a desire to fight the commands of the hypnotist." Structuring the suggestions to align with client goals will be most effective. (*Example*: "You will feel proud that you have made a decision to stop smoking (lose weight). You will follow my suggestions because you choose, because you desire. No one can make you do anything against your will, only when you choose.")

Care should always be taken when structuring hypnotic suggestion to use ego-developing images and ideas. Negative suggestions tend to be short-term in their impact and wear off quickly. It is difficult to motivate people to reinforce suggestions that are unpleasant for them; we instinctively seek pleasure. Positive suggestions will have a greater impact and are more likely to be adopted by the client. (*Example*: "You will notice that food will taste better to you as your senses clear from the effect of cigarettes." *Not* "You will become nauseated whenever you light a cigarette.").

Hypnotic suggestion during the induction should be directed toward all the areas of the habit that were found to be problematic during the assessment phase. For example, if the therapist has learned that motivation is marginal, then the hypnotic suggestions should be strongly directed to bolstering the desire to change. If specific trigger situations were identified during the assessment process, then direct and indirect hypnotic suggestions will be used to intervene in the unconscious conditioned response.

Length of Treatment

The client should be encouraged to arrange the hypnosis intervention for the point in time when they are prepared to cease smoking. If a smoking client strongly desires a period of time in which to switch brands or cut down, he or she should be encouraged to postpone the hypnosis intervention until after this period has been completed.

Weight-loss clients tend to desire large amounts of weight loss in a very brief period of time. However, the goal of a good weight-loss program should be to help the client make longterm permanent changes in eating habits and approach to food. It is important for the therapist to state and restate this goal of longterm permanent change, and to help the client realize that eating habits acquired over a lifetime cannot be changed overnight. Setting a long-range timeline will be helpful because weight loss will usually be gradual and erratic. It will be helpful if the client realizes this as part of the treatment regime. (*Example*: "Picture yourself the way you would like to look. You know that this is a goal that you can achieve, you know that you will be able to work every day toward achieving your goal.")

---

*See Chapter 3.

The number of sessions that are anticipated should be specified. For smoking-control clients an initial session in which the intervention is structured and implemented, and a follow-up session approximately two week later, are usually sufficient. Success rate tends to be high in the first two weeks following a hypnotic intervention, with the dropoff beginning after that period. The client should be encouraged to return for the second session to provide a longterm reinforcement of the suggestions.

Weight-loss clients should anticipate needing regularly scheduled hypnosis sessions until they reach their goal. For clients with only 10 pounds to lose, one session with follow-up and a reinforcement cassette tape may suffice. However, clients with significant amounts of weight to lose will need to return for periodic reinforcement of the suggestions in addition to using their cassette tapes twice daily.

Integrating Other Inteventions

Results of a hypnosis intervention for weight or smoking control will be greatly improved if the session is structured so that hypnosis is used as part of a holistic intervention plan. Vick, Dubin, and Beder (1983) studied 3000 people who were treated in holistic American Lung Association program, which gave clients information about the effects of smoking, provided group hypnosis treatment, and offered a variety of support systems. A one-year follow-up study showed 44 percent of the respondents were still not smoking. This holistic model provides the client with support and information needed as well as the hypnotic intervention that will increase the likelihood of success.

Reinforcement

The client should be advised of the importance of reinforcement of the hypnotic suggestions. This may take the form of a cassette tape of the hypnotic induction. There is a direct correlation between success of a hypnosis program and use of a reinforcement tape. Smokers should be advised to use their tape at least twice daily during the first two weeks. Weight-control clients should be advised to listen to their tape twice daily until they reach their desired weight goal. For clients in longterm weight-loss programs, it is helpful for the therapist to have a series of tapes available because the same tape can become tedious after a period of time. The reinforcement tape should be two-sided, approximately 10 to 12 minutes per side, and should highlight the hypnotic suggestions used during the session.

Evaluation and Follow-Up

Follow-up is an important aspect of any habit-change intervention. Habits are generally deeply ingrained. Initial success and high motivation will often be followed by periods of disillusionment. During these times the client is likely to revert to the old behavior patterns unless some kind of support and ongoing structure are available.

Smoking clients will often be initially successful with one hypnosis session and the cassette tape for reinforcement. This initial success will tend to last from two weeks to three months. However, during the first highly stressful life event encountered after quitting, clients will often experience a reemergence of the desire to smoke, by the desire to have "just one cigarette" or to smoke "only" during the time of the stress and then quit again. Once the behavior pattern begins, however, it will tend to continue. For this reason, the therapist should include follow-up at regular intervals throughout the first nonsmoking year as part of the treatment plan. The client should understand that this follow-up will serve to reinforce nonsmoking behaviors and remove the behaviors that may have begun to reemerge. (It is important in planning follow-up that the therapist *not* imply that the client will begin smoking again, as this can act as a suggestion of failure).

Weight-loss clients will generally need frequent and repeated follow-up until they reach their goal weight and for a period of time beyond. The habit of overeating is difficult to change, and clients will routinely experience periods of slow weight loss or none. They will often become discouraged and give up. Ongoing sessions every two to four weeks will serve to maintain desire and motivation. These sessions can easily be conducted in a group. This allows sharing of the experience and development of support and structure mechanisms.

SUGGESTED READING

Sidis, B. (1898). *The psychology of suggestion.* New York: D. Appleton, pp. 10–23.

Spiegel, H., & Spiegel, D. (1978). *Trance and treatment.* New York: Basic Books, pp. 165–188.

Stunkard, A. (1983). Biological and psychological factors in obesity. In Goodstein, R. (Ed.) *Eating and weight disorders.* New York: Springer Publishing.

Vick, C., Dubin, B., & Beder, B. (1983). A multidisciplinary approach to smoking withdrawal in ongoing economical and successful community-based programs. Proceedings of the *Fifth World Conference on Smoking and Health.* Winnipeg, Canada, p. 181.

REFERENCES

Browning, M. (1974). *The nursing process in practice* New York: American Journal of Nursing Company.

Erickson, M., Rossi, E., & Rossi, S. (1976). *Hypnotic realities.* New York: Irvington Publishers.

Fenichel, O. (1945). *The psychoanalytic theory of neurosis.* New York: W.W. Norton.

Fritschler, A. (1975). *Smoking and politics.* Englewood Cliffs, NJ: Prentice-Hall.

Goodstein, R. (1979). *Eating and weight disorders.* New York: Parthenon Books.

Kalkman, M., & Davis, A. (1974). *New dimensions in mental health-psychiatric nursing.* New York: McGraw-Hill.

Mennies, J.M. (1983). Smoking, the physiologic effects. *American Journal of Nursing,* 8, 1143–1146.

National Cancer Institute. (1981). Calling it quits. (*N.I.H. publication 81-1824.*) Bethesda, MD: Office of Cancer Communications.

Totman, R. (1979). *Social causes of illness.* New York: Parthenon Books.

Winter, R. (1980). *The scientific case against smoking.* New York: Crown Publishers.

13

Metaphor and Indirect Suggestion in the Treatment of Recovering Alcoholics*

Stanley Meyers

Recovery from alcoholism is a developmental process, proceeding through stages analogous to those of ego development (Mahler, Pine, & Bergman, 1975) and requiring interventions appropriate to the patient's stage of recovery.

The intoxicated alcoholic patient presents to the hospital in an "autistic" state during which the treatment staff must provide all support: medical, emotional, and physical. Typically the patient is detoxified using one of a variety of drugs such as benzodiazepoxides or phenobarbital, which cross-tolerate with the alcohol and ease the withdrawal symptoms. In this stage, the patient is totally dependent on the staff and any attempts at standard psychotherapy are at best wasted and at worst alienating.

Following detoxification, the patient enters the "early symbiotic" phase of recovery. In this stage the staff must still provide considerable support and lend many ego functions: stimulus barrier, judgment, reasoning, reality testing, regulation and control of affects, impulses, drives, and interpersonal relationships (Bellak, Gediman, & Hurvich, 1973). The patient is now able to communicate and learn some basics, such as the concept of Alcoholics Anonymous (A.A.) and group interaction. He or she may also be introduced to disulfiram (Antabuse) and taught the essentials of nutrition. Although alcoholics

---

*Editor's note: This chapter describes indirect and metaphoric approaches with the alcoholic. The background and theory is described in the Ericksonian section of Chapter 2 and in the section on indirect suggestions in Chapter 3. Because these are more subtle forms of intervention the editor recommends that the reader attend to those chapters before reading this chapter.

are different from young children in their ability to use language at this point, they may still be emotionally unable to process verbal data directly and meaningfully. Indirect suggestions, metaphors, and fantasy/imagery serve as more adequate vehicles for learning. These communications are phase-appropriate and maturational nutrients which can be emotionally digested without causing the painful upset of premature interpretation (Ormont & Strean, 1978).

The next phase of recovery is a transition from the hospital into outpatient group and individual counseling and psychotherapy. Early outpatient treatment is analogous to the middle and late stages of symbiosis, in which the child starts to differentiate self from mother and enters a practicing subphase of trying life out, with the comfort of returning to the nest for recharging in a rapprochement subphase.

The recovering alcoholic is best served by the therapist realizing that the patient has different maturational needs at various stages of recovery and *cannot* be treated with standard dynamic therapy in early recovery as if sober for years (Ormont & Strean, 1978). Biologically the brain is recovering from the physical trauma of the alcohol abuse, and psychologically the ego's task is to recover from the emotional and social damage of drinking.

This chapter describes some techniques used with recovering alcoholics in an inpatient hospital setting, an outpatient alcoholism clinic, and private practice. The patients are both dual diagnosed alcoholics (those with borderline and psychotic illness) and those with alcoholism alone.

STRATEGIES AND TACTICS FOR INTERVENTION

Many issues complicate the treatment of alcoholics. These patients often want immediate results and try to accomplish too many changes all at once. Ego strength, impulse control, and judgment are often minimal in early recovery. Slips (relapses) are therefore not uncommon on the road to sobriety. The problems of engaging the patient and of counter-transference complicate treatment.

One of the first hurdles the alcoholism therapist must overcome is despair at having a room full of patients who do not talk to the therapist or to each other except in a superficial way. They withdraw and isolate themselves, frustrating the therapist with their "I'm all right, Jack" attitude. Their apparent and easily labeled resistance is metaphorically expressed in physical acting-out around coffee and cigarettes. The leader can introduce an indirect suggestion such as, "Even though you don't want to stop smoking, you will find you have much better things to give each other (yourselves)." This is both an embedded command (Erickson & Rossi, 1979) and a metaphor about interpersonal relatedness and can be readily transposed to a stop-drinking directive. An embedded command is an indirect suggestion placed in a sentence in such a way that the apparent message hides the real command. The example above has a different meaning if read this way: "Even though you don't want to . . . *stop smoking (drinking)*." The template for this type of embedded command is the Ericksonian hypnotic suggestion, "Even though you don't want to go into a trance now. . . ." While the conscious mind is waiting for the end of the sentence, the unconscious mind, which doesn't process negatives, receives the command, "Go into a trance, *now!*"

These techniques are more workable than the use of intellectual appeals and interpretations with patients in early recovery from alcoholism.

A Basic Strategy: Metaphor

A metaphor is the figurative use of a word, phrase, or story in place of another to suggest an analogy between them. Therapeutic metaphors involve fantasy and/or imagery and the use of metaphor is a strategy; the specific metaphors used are tactics to help bring about change. Metaphors bypass conscious protective maneuvers, which is especially useful in treating alcoholics, who often use denial, intellectualization, and avoidance. In psychotherapy metaphors can be auditory (verbal), visual (pictoral), or kinesthetic (movement-based). When selecting a metaphor, it is crucial to match the preferred mode of the patient (Bandler & Grinder, 1975). A typical pitfall for the beginning therapist (and not a few experienced ones) is to use the metaphoric mode favored by the therapist without regard for the patient's preferred way of accessing and processing information. To illustrate this point, I might start this paragraph in at least four different ways:

1. To illustrate this point or to give you a clear *picture* (visual metaphor).
2. I'd like to make this point as *clear as a bell*, so you will have no trouble *hearing* me (auditory metaphor).
3. I want you to get a *gut feeling* for what I've spent years getting *a handle on* (kinesthetic metaphor).
4. I'd like you to get the *taste and smell* of these *savory* techniques (olfactory/gustatory metaphor).

Bandler & Grinder (1975) gave a detailed description of how to ascertain accessing/processing modes from observation of eye movements. A simpler and less exact way is to simply listen to the patient and hear or observe, get a feeling for, or get a whiff or taste of his or her preferred mode. This precaution must be taken seriously, or the therapist runs the risk of at best not communicating, and at worst creating a resistance that needn't exist. For example, I once suggested that an early recovering alcoholic patient change seats and speak to an empty chair (Perls, 1969), a standard Gestalt therapy technique. The patient refused and I persisted, insisting this would be "helpful" to him. He gave me excellent supervision by suggesting that I find a way of dealing with him that "sounded better" and was more congenial to his style. When I switched to a purely auditory and noninterpretive mode, he was more able to "hear" me, of course. The moral of the story is in an old proverb. It's easier to ride a horse in the direction it is going.

Tactics: Exercises and Fantasy/Imagery Techniques

The following interventions are useful exercises for alcoholics in early recovery. These can be practiced by students before implementing them with patients.

One Step at a Time

This A.A. motto counters the obsessional and impulse-ridden alcoholic's desire to prematurely do things for which he or she is not prepared, or to suddenly go from a poorly worked-through intellectualization to major life change, for instance:

- "Okay, Doc, so now that I'm sober and I know that my fear of intimacy is keeping me away from women, I'm going to go out and marry the first lady who is agreeable" (impulsive).
- "So now I'm sober and I know about my fear of intimacy as the source of my loneliness and my drinking, but nothing changes, so what good is therapy anyway? I might as well drink!" (obsessional).

To counter these impulses, the patient is asked to stand at one side of the room and instructed to broad-jump to the farthest clear spot in the room. Usually the patient gets four to five feet in a jump, and the therapist directs the patient to try again. After a few tries (and it is important to encourage the patient to keep trying), the patient usually gives up. He or she is then directed to take one slow step at a time, saying with each step, "only a fool (jerk, dope, etc.) does it one step at a time." When the patient reaches the other side of the room, the therapist asks, "Where are you now? How long did it take you to get there? How long would it have taken you the other way?" The patient is addressing his/her resistance by calling it "stupid." "One step at a time" is the desired outcome. This exercise is a kinesthetic (action oriented) metaphor for the repetition compulsion. The repetition compulsion is a valiant attempt to repeat over and over the unsuccessful past solutions, using the same old tools that never worked before. "So what?" you may ask. "Couldn't you just tell the patient what he or she is doing and explain or direct a better way?"

Rather than answer, I'll suggest another game,* which can be played by two patients in a group. One takes the role of the patient (P) and the other the therapist (T). At the end the roles are reversed and the game replayed. P is to

---

*Games are defined as formal sets of operations with a goal, not as trivial or demeaning operations.

tell T about his or her difficulty in getting things done all at once. T first interprets to P that this is a repetition of P's desire to please his or her parents through premature ego functioning (an accurate but useless intervention early on in treatment) and that P can now learn to do things in a more orderly and phase-appropriate manner. P and T are to pause for a moment and feel the emotional impact of this intervention. Then T is to instruct P to do the "one-step" (broad-jump) exercise, and experience this learning kinesthetically.

This procedure can be practiced first by two students taking the role of patient and therapist. This dyadic role playing would best be used after each metaphor so that the student can experience the role of P in a given therapy mode and find out in a practical rather than theoretical way his or her own preferred learning mode.

Doing it the Hard Way

Neurotic behavior in general and alcoholic behavior specifically are unnecessary activity and fruitless expenditure of energy toward often unrealistic goals. Again, some kinesthetic metaphors quickly demonstrate the futility of such behavior. The following exercises symbolize the many failed "home remedies" alcoholics try before entering treatment:

- Ask the patient to pick up a chair by grasping the lowermost portion of one leg. (Hardly anyone can do this, but almost anyone can pick up the chair by holding it by the back.)
- Ask the patient to stand up and imagine a 50-pound rock is falling straight down on him or her. Then ask the patient to imagine catching it—not likely, but slightly possible. Ask how hard it would be to simply step aside. Then ask, would it be any harder to step aside if the rock weighed 1,000 pounds.
- Another kinesthetic metaphor is about people who are so inefficient and circuitous that they scratch their left ear with their right hand. This is particularly useful for alcoholics, who tend to be negative and pseudoindependent ("I want to do it my own way"). The therapist can instruct the patient to scratch his or her left ear by placing the right hand (1) behind the head, (2) under the left arm, (3) under the left or right leg, (4) the most difficult way possible. This form of intervention must be done carefully and respectfully to avoid any intimation that is ridiculing the patient. If the patient says something such as, "Are you making fun of me?" or "Are you laughing at me?" The therapist can say, "I am trying to help you to experience your behavior in a way that's meaningful to you. You are not laughable to me. What is your own response to the behavior you see?"

It is particularly important to be very gentle with paranoid and borderline patients and alcoholics, who early in recovery easily feel ridiculed and ashamed. If the therapist takes a serious and respectful attitude toward the patient and the exercises, negative reactions are minimized.

Beating One's Head Against A Wall

The most powerful alcoholism treatment modality is A.A., whose philosophy encompasses 12 steps. The first step in A.A.'s program of recovery from alcoholism is "We admitted we were powerless over alcohol—that our lives had become unmanageable." This profound step is illustrated in the following metaphor/fantasy, used with patients who complain of how hard and how long they are struggling with little success:

> Imagine that you are standing in front of a brick wall and banging your head against the wall trying to break through. It has now been many years and you are bloodied, but the wall has not budged. You valiantly continue, even increasing your efforts, never giving up. Now imagine that 20 feet down the wall there is an open archway. What would you have to do to see it? First you would have to stop banging your head (admit powerlessness), second, wipe the blood out of your eyes, third, step back, turn your head and look.

This visual and kinesthetic metaphor vividly illustrates the necessary preconditions for taking the first step. In ego psychology terms, there is the abatement of superego attacks (self-criticism), clear acceptance of what is in reality happening (reality testing), and assessment of alternative possibilities (judgment, reasoning, etc.)

Relive the Slip

Basic to recovery is acceptance of and surrender to the disease of alcoholism. Reluctance to admit this powerlessness, to live one day at a time, and to take one step at a time ironically ends in return to drinking—the alcoholic "slip."

Alcoholics often are mystified by their transition from nondrinking to drinking states. For instance, a hospitalized 30-year-old male told the following story of his last drinking bout:

> I was just walking down the street, going to an A.A. meeting. I was just 90 days sober. It was a beautiful day, and suddenly nature called, just as I was passing my favorite bar. So I hooked a left into the bar, waved at the bartender, who beckoned me over, so what could I do? I didn't want to be impolite, so I went over to the bar to say hello. Well, lo and behold, he had my favorite drink on the bar. So what could I do? I drank it, so as not to be rude, and I just kept on drinking.

The patient was encouraged to stand up and renarrate the story, taking one brief step at a time, and at each critical juncture (e.g., left turn into bar, going up to the bar, taking the drink), he was asked to fully fill in his thoughts, feelings, and possible alternative actions that would have maintained sobriety. In short, he was asked to experience various ego functions: delay of gratification, judgment, reasoning, and reality testing in place of impulsive behavior. He could have been asked to replay the scene in various ways to bring it to a different (and sober) conclusion.

Talk to the Bottle

Grieving the loss of alcohol is a necessary step in the alcoholic's recovery. In this exercise, the therapist places a liquor bottle on a chair in front of the patients' asking the patient to talk to the bottle and tell it all of the good things alcohol did for him. If the patient can't or won't verbalize any, the therapist can suggest the following: social facilitation, anxiety reduction, overcoming shyness, no one ever met a bottle that said "no" to them, etc. This exercise can be done individually or as a group exercise. It also can be done in a more elaborate form as "The Funeral for Al. K. Hall." The therapist sets up a fantasy/imagery situation of a funeral where the deceased is "your old friend, Al K. Hall." Then each of the "mourners" (group members) is to eulogize their old friend.

The basic point of both these exercises is that alcohol use was at first a partly successful attempt at self-medication and reparation. The alcoholic must learn to accept the loss of the positive effects of alcohol and mourn them in order to truly develop a more adaptive means of coping with problems. The therapist must carefully keep the mourners from making negative statements as these block the expression of the positive ones, which are the point of the exercise.

The Bottle in the Middle of the Road

For many alcoholics, the "bottle" is an overshadowing presence in their conscious, preconscious, and unconscious lives, directly or indirectly blocking their progress. In this exercise, the patients are helped into an imagery state with the following statement.

> Close your eyes and pay attention to your breathing and my words. Don't try to clear your mind, but allow any thoughts that come in to enter, play out on the screen of your mind, and leave. Don't try to keep them out, don't try to stop them, and don't try to keep them from leaving. Now, little by little, as your breathing becomes deeper and more regular, and your body relaxes and your mind clears, I'd like you to imagine yourself walking along a narrow mountain road on a bright sunny day when suddenly you notice a giant bottle of booze in the middle of the road, with impassable boulders on either side.

The patients are first asked to verbalize their fantasies and feelings about meeting the bottle unexpectedly and then to talk about how they feel being blocked by it. They are then encouraged to imagine ways around the bottle, over it, through it, or under it. The type of fantasy created is diagnostic of each patient's state of mind. Some patients just give up, some call on others to help, some climb up on a ladder to see over the bottle, some try to break it, etc.

The point of this exercise is twofold: first, to bring to awareness and to the realm of conscious ego functioning the unconscious fantasy that the bottle is blocking their progress, and, second, to allow the patient an opportunity to struggle with and overcome the unconscious block. Among the solutions patients invented are pushing over the bottle and swimming through the spilled liquor and using the overturned bottle as a sled down the mountain.

Plan Your Next Drunk

Bateson (1972) stated that alcoholics cannot, or do not, think through the consequences of their future drinking, instead trying to avoid drinking by willpower and not thinking about drinking. He pointed out that sobriety returns the alcoholic to the conditions that drove him or her to drink in the first place. The notion that he or she has overcome alcohol is exactly what allows the alcoholic to become less vigilant and to "slip."

The following exercise usually elicits resistance and often anger from recovering alcoholics. It's called, "Plan your next drunk." The patients are asked to plan, in vivid and minute detail, each step of their next drunk, what they are going to drink, where they are going to get it, how they are going to serve it, with whom, where, when, how, under what emotional conditions, and what the consequences will be. This strengthens ego functioning by allowing full verbalization of the imagined circumstances *without* action. It is most important to assure patients that thinking and talking about drinking is not the same as drinking. Indeed, this is one basic definition of the ego function of reality testing.

Guilt Reduction

The fourth and fifth steps of A.A. are:

4. Made a searching and fearless moral inventory of ourselves.
5. Admitted to God, to ourselves, and to another human being the exact nature of our wrongs.

In order to take these steps, a patient must first reduce his or her guilt to a manageable level or the awareness of self-responsibility will be too painful. There are several methods for accomplishing this goal.

The first method derives from the work of Gibbons (1979). The patient is put into a trance and then told, using metaphor, that the guilt he or she feels is excessive and out of proportion to anything the patient may ever have done. These metaphors suggest that it is time to let go of the guilt and that the patient can do so in good conscience. The second method is for the patient to imagine being wrapped in cotton batting so that the effect of criticism by oneself or another is insulated by the material. In the third method, the patient imagines spinning a special cocoon that is transparent and semipermeable, so only what the patient can handle emotionally is allowed in.

These techniques abate the attack of primitive superego attitudes on the emergent ego of the recovering alcoholic, allowing the ego to grow and develop in a nonhostile atmosphere.

Conflict: To Drink or Not to Drink

The Jungian concept of subpersonae making up the personality (Jung, 1938) can be applied to alcoholism treatment. This method of conflict resolution and problem solving derived originally from psychodrama (Moreno, 1946), and Gestalt therapy (Perls, 1969). The patient plays the role of the part of them that wants to drink, and the part that doesn't. The dramatization of mother and father and any significant others and their attitudes toward alcohol and the patient are other applications of this Jungian concept. This can be done individually, with the patient changing chairs for each role, or in a group with members coached to play some of the roles. The therapist encourages a dialogue among the personae so that all of the patient's thoughts, feelings, fantasies, wishes, and impulses are put into words. In this dialogue, the therapist actively prompts the various personae in their roles and statements: defending alcohol, rejecting alcohol, criticizing, apologizing, etc. All of the warded-off and denied impulses are placed under the aegis of ego functioning through verbalization. This technique allows for verbalization and examination of patient's introjected and often unconscious parental attitudes.

CONCLUSION

The techniques described are useful with clients suffering from various clinical entities, not only alcoholism. They illustrate in a vivid and immediate way sound metapsychological and developmental concepts, and a method of delivering interpretations that is not harmful to the ego-impaired patient. These techniques can be quite powerful and evocative, and must be used, like all interventions, with a clear view of the patient's diagnosis, state of anxiety, level of confusion, and ability to tolerate the intervention.

These techniques are not done for their own sake, nor for mere drama nor for unintegrated catharsis. In short, use them sparingly, carefully, tactfully, and be prepared to drop the game and change the subject of conversation if the patient exhibits undue resistance, confusion, or distress. Such reactions do not necessarily mean that the patient is opposing you or that you are doing anything wrong. What they do suggest is that either the timing or the metaphor itself is inappropriate for the particular patient. Finally, remember that these methods are vehicles, not laws, and are meant to suggest possibilities for you to invent your own metaphors and games. The goal is to vividly illustrate to patients what it is essential for them to understand.

REFERENCES

Bandler, R., & Grinder, J. (1975). *The structure of magic*. Palo Alto, CA: Science and Behavior Books.

Bateson, G. (1972). *Steps to an ecology of mind*. New York: Ballantine Books.

Bellak, L., Gediman, H.K., & Hurvich, M. (1973). *Ego functions in schizophrenics, neurotics, and normals*. New York: John Wiley.

Erickson, M.H., & Rossi, E. (1979). *Hypnotherapy: An exploratory casebook*. New York: Irvington Publishers.

Gibbons, D.R. (1979). *Applied hypnosis and hyperempiria*. New York: Plenum Press.

Jung, C.G. (1938). *The basic writings*. New York: Random House, Modern Library.

Mahler, M.S., Pine, F., & Bergman, A. (1975). *The psychological birth of the human infant*. New York: Basic Books.

Moreno, J.L. (1946). *Psychodrama*. New York: Beacon House.

Ormont, L.R., & Strean, H.S. (1978). *The practice of conjoint therapy*. New York: Human Science Press.

Perls, F.S. (1969). *Gestalt therapy verbatim*. Moab, UT: Real People Press.

14

Treatment of Hypertension: Two Case Studies

Rothlyn P. Zahourek[*]

Hypertension has been referred to as a "silent killer" because most individuals with hypertension appear healthy and experience few symptoms. Yet when blood pressure is elevated to only 140/90 mm Hg, a risk for premature death exists. In today's society, hypertension is a common health problem, affecting over 40 million Americans. When pharmacology is the only method of treatment, young and middle-aged adults may expect to remain on medication for 30 to 40 years (Wadden & de la Torre, 1980), a discouraging prospect. If side effects such as drowsiness, fatigue, impotence, and depression occur, patients become less willing to take medication. As a result, many are noncompliant with medical treatment.

PHYSIOLOGY

Sustained hypertension results in fibrinoid necrosis of the arterioles, most often in the brain and kidney. The necrotic tissue is replaced by fibrinous material that causes small hemorrhages and clots in the weakened arteriole walls (Taylor & Fortman, 1983).

Blood pressure was traditionally believed to be influenced by neural networks and chemical and hormonal mechanisms that affect the walls of the

---

*Case example "Bernice" written by Marcia Fishman.

195

vascular system. The autonomic nervous sytem largely regulates blood pressure, reacting to emotional stimuli and to higher cerebral functions. Anatomically, blood pressure reacts to muscle tension in the body through the simple mechanics of constricting blood vessels. There are, however, multiple factors involved, as individuals with normal peripheral resistance may become hypertensive. Furthermore, in addition to physiology, familial and environmental factors must be considered (Falkner, Onesti, & Hamstra, 1981). Increased blood pressure is now seen as a symptom rather than a disease itself and should be understood from a systems point of view. Single-cause explanations are insufficient as various systems seem to interact to produce pressure changes, and intervention must take into account the interplay of these systems (Harburg, Blakelock, & Roger, 1973).

While controversial, two physiologic mechanisms are thought to be responsible for hypertension: The renin–angiotension aldosterone axis regulates arterial pressure and sodium balance. Hypertension results from vasoconstriction and blood volume. Excess renin causes vasoconstriction, and excess volume is related to aldosteronism.

Guyton (1980) argued that only the renal body-fluid control mechanism has the ability to return blood pressure to normal. The nervous system, however, has continued to be viewed as playing a major role in blood pressure (Taylor and Fortman, 1983):

- Sympathetic activity affects blood pressure volume by directly affecting the kidney. Increased sympathetic activity can precipitate kidney failure; change in the glomerular filtration rate leads to increased sodium reabsorption.
- Animals who receive drugs producing generalized sympathectomy have profound blood pressure drop.
- Sympathetic activity is altered with some hypertension. Norepinephrine increases significantly during exercise in hypertensives. In patients with labile hypertension, elevated catecholamines are consistently found.

Neural (emotional) factors may initiate, maintain, or exacerbate hypertension (Taylor & Fortman, 1983).

Psychosocial variables have also become increasingly considered. Stress and loss are commonly associated with hypertension (Benson, 1977; D'Artri & Ostfeld, 1975; Grahm, 1945; Henry & Cassel, 1969; Reiser, 1951; Kasl, Cobb, 1970). Psychogenic, personality, and neurogenic factors have similarly been argued over the years. Alexander and colleagues (1968) hypothesized that hypertension is related to repressed anger and the inability to be assertive, which lead to tension and constricted peripheral blood vessels. Barbara Brown (1977) contended that the hypertensive wants to strike back but cannot. She recommended stress-reducing techniques and assertiveness training to help the individual relax, live more effectively, and subsequently reduce blood pressure. More recent research (Weiner, 1977; Harrell, 1980) does not support the early personality theories that hypertensive patients have a particular personality. Others, (Harburg, et al., 1979) however, found that hypertensive patients have difficulty expressing feelings— particularly anger—to others and that stress is an important element in their lives.

In reviewing the current research on hypertension, Taylor and Fortman (1983) stated that while these theories have not consistently been found to be significantly related to hypertension, they warrant consideration when planning treatment. Since hypertensives do not seem to like anger, helping them cope with intense feelings and with a general sense of well-being is in order.

We know that highly stimulating imagery produces cardiovascular changes. May and Johnson (1973) reported increased heart rate associated with stimulating images, and Sheikh et al. (1979) reported that imagery can modify blood pressure, heart rate, and oxygen consumption. Calm peaceful imagery has been associated with relaxation and dilated blood vessels resulting in skin temperature changes (Brown, 1977).

Many techniques have been used to manage hypertension, including Benson's "relaxation response," Jacobsen's progressive relaxation, autogenic training, transcendental meditation, Buddhist meditation, galvanic skin response biofeedback, blood pressure biofeedback, and hypnosis. Wadden and de la Torre (1980) reviewed these methods in the following categories:

1. Methods that focused on the subject's elicitation of deep muscle relaxation
2. Techniques that produced a meditational state characterized by a reduced respiratory rate
3. Hypnotic approaches
4. Approaches that used biofeedback instrumentation with instructions to lower blood pressure

They found subjects, whether taking medications or not, were significantly able to reduce blood pressure when using muscle relaxation. In those not using medication, subjects were able to reduce their systolic readings between 7 and 14.8 mm Hg. In the studies using hypnosis, the subjects were induced into deep physical relaxation through suggestions of muscle heaviness and relaxing imagery. Direct suggestions to relax internal organs, including the circulatory system, were also given. Some reports document success equal to progressive relaxation and meditation (Deabler, 1973; Friedman & Taub, 1978) while others do not (Lane & Ruskin, 1950). In one case, hypnosis produced small but significant increases in blood pressure (Case, Fogel, & Pollack, 1980). This study deserves some additional discussion. First, the sample size was small (15 subjects). Small but significant rises in blood pressure (pressor effect) occurred during the inductions and while practicing self-hypnosis. After four months the elevation was maintained by three patients, while five patients with the highest initial diastolic pressure had reduced their pressures. Hypnotizable subjects with the lowest initial pressures exhibited the pressor effect. All fifteen reported an increased sense of well-being and behavior changes. Speigel's (1974) induction techqniue was utilized, and although the goal is relaxation and positive suggestion, the technique demands concentration and some degree of performance from the subject. This in itself might have caused the pressor effect, and further study comparing different methods of induction is needed.

Wadden and de la Torre (1980) emphasized that the studies using hypnosis suffer from many methodological difficulties, including (1) lack of baseline data, (2) absence of random assignment ot treatment groups, and (3) failure to control attention adequately.

Studies utilizing biofeedback have shown significant results, but questions remain about long term effectiveness and the influence of expensive equipment on practical widespread use. These results do not show a statistically significant difference between relaxation and biofeedback, but relaxation techniques seem to have a slight edge (Wadden & de la Torre, 1980).

When treatment is planned, numerous factors must be considered: salt intake, weight, environmental situations, lifestyle, personal behavioral patterns, stress, and emotions. Rest and relaxation, appropriate handling of anger and stress, and medications are commonly recommended.

The introduction to the June, 1980 issue of *Behavioral Medicine* summarized the important aspects of hypertension:

1. The hypertensive patient often experiences anxiety, doubt, inadequacy, and fear about the future.
2. Compliance differs markedly depending on the physician, the patient, and the therapeutic protocol, including medication, biofeedback, meditation, relaxation, imagery, and hypnosis.
3. Behavioral therapy approaches are generally not adequate to manage the disease, but can be a valuable adjunct to treatment.

Sufficiently documented results are common enough for nurses to use hypnotic techniques and hypnosis when caring for hypertensive patients. Most often techqniues are combined with medication. Medical management, monitoring, and collaborating with the physician are imperative.

The following are dramatically different case examples. One, a medical emergency, by the secondary author, occurred in an acute general hospital setting, while the other occurred in an outpatient private psychotherapy practice situation. The latter case by the primary author involved supportive psychotherapy and general stress management as well as techniques specifically related to blood pressure reduction.

Case Example: Acute Crisis

Bernice, a 42-year-old black woman, had been mildly hypertensive before her pregnancy. She admittedly did not follow the physician's medical regimen. Her state of expectancy was enough of an added burden to push her into toxemia.

Her noncompliance was in part due to the fact she only had a fourth-grade education. She found most of our written instructions far too complex to understand. However, her lack of formal education did not interfere with her ability to use hypnotic techniques during the crisis.

Bernice had an emergency caesarean section because of the toxemia. Even after the delivery of a healthy child and the use of various antihypertensive drugs, her blood pressure remained dangerously high (300/198 mm Hg!). She was seriously ill and very frightened. When we first met she had not slept in several days. Though very tired, she was extremely agitated and complained of an excruciating headache. She told me she felt as if her head would burst. The health care team feared Bernice could have a massive stroke and die. One of her physicians asked if I would be willing to try hypnosis. For the past 12 hours all of her medications had been stopped because of their ineffectiveness.

When the physician and I went into her room we found Bernice sitting at the edge of the bed. She was attached to an ECG monitor, and had an IV, an arterial line, a central venous pressure line, and a Foley catheter in place. I introduced myself and told her I had a way to make her feel much more comfortable. I told her "the relaxation" exercises would not hurt and were similar to those she had been taught in her prenatal classes. She was willing to try anything, but only if she could sit in a chair. I said yes, while at the same time the physician said, "no!' I held firm, quietly stating there was no reason Bernice could not be in the large easy chair, and it would enhance the procedure by giving Bernice some control over her immediate situation. We assisted her into the chair. She asked if I was going to make her all better and I told her I was interested in helping her feel better. She seemed to understand, although her thoughts were somewhat confused. (Because of the severe hypertension, it was surprising she could think at all.) I was concerned about her being able to focus sufficiently on my suggestions, but everyone involved felt it was worth a try. Bernice was sitting upright and extremely tense. She said any movement hurt her head more.

I told Bernice that if I asked her to do anything she found uncomfortable, she could change it herself or ask me to alter the suggestion. I asked her to close her eyes as it would make her less dizzy. Then I had her breathe in and out slowly. I suggested as she did that she would feel calmer and quieter. After several minutes we noticed a smile on her face. Her respirations were slower and deeper, and she indicated by nodding that she felt calmer.

I decided to use progressive relaxation since this was familiar to her from the prenatal classes. I began by asking her to tighten and release the muscles in her toes: first curling them and then relaxing them, then flexing her feet, etc. However, something very strange happened. She did nothing with her feet. Instead she grimaced her face tightly and then relaxed. She didn't respond when I asked her if anything was wrong. At this moment the physician, who was watching the monitors, motioned to me. Her ECG was slower and regular and her blood pressure was down to 290/185 mm Hg.

I decided to continue giving suggestions to systematically tense and relax the various muscle groups, working up the body. Bernice continue to do just the opposite, working *down* her body. (Remember whenever using these techniques, it is the patient/client who maintains control, not the therapist.) She was physically showing signs of becoming more relaxed. She was now leaning back in the chair looking more comfortable. Her ECG showed normal sinus rhythm and a rate of 68 to 70 beats/min. (When we started her pulse had been 110 with intermittent premature beats.) Over 30 minutes her blood pressure came down to 275/180 mm Hg. Someone dropped a tray outside her room, yet there was no observable response. However, when I asked her to breathe in and out more rapidly, she did so. I asked her to raise and lower her right hand, which she did. I now gave the suggestion of her lying in a warm tub of water, just relaxing and feeling calmer and more comfortable. When I asked, she said her headache was going away.

I suggested she remain in the tub a while longer, then I would count to three and she would open her eyes and feel much better. Her blood pressure was now holding at 260/150. Certainly not perfect, but much better. Just as important, Bernice *felt* better.

The physician motioned to me that he wanted her brought out of the trance state. It was approximately 40 minutes from the time we started. I slowly counted to three. I asked her to open her eyes. Nothing. Again, I counted to three and asked her to open her eyes. Still, nothing. Then I realized that Bernice was asleep! Over the next two hours her blood pressure continued decreasing to 190/140 mm Hg and she slept soundly. When she woke up almost two hours later she looked and felt much better. She still had a headache, but a "dull one." She wasn't dizzy anymore. It was obvious she was not agitated or as frightened.

Marci: Bernice, do you remember what I was saying to you?

Bernice: Oh, yes!

Marci: Would you answer some questions for me?

Bernice: Sure.

Marci: When I asked you to tighten and relax your muscles from your feet up, you were doing it from the head down. Would you tell me why?

Bernice: (Tears in her eyes, she quietly explained.) I was afraid I was going to die. I knew I was very sick. Do you know the old saying, "Having your feet planted firmly on the ground"? I knew if I kept my feet firmly on the floor I would be okay. That's why I had to sit in the chair. I knew you wouldn't mind. But the doc gets mad.

Bernice made me realize how important it was for patients to have control over their own lives, and that the therapist will be most successful when permissive, knowing that all behavior has meaning.

Marci: Bernice, when I counted to three and asked you to open your eyes, did you hear me?

Bernice: Oh yes, I heard you just fine. But this was the first time I felt better in so long I knew it was safe to go to sleep.

I saw Bernice again later that evening, only this time she followed my suggestions fully. She trusted me and herself. I suggested she do the exercises herself. We discussed how and when she would do her relaxation and imagery exercises. Her husband and 16-year-old daughter even learned to help her. Bernice and I worked at getting her pressure down. While in the hospital her blood pressure decreased to 190/100 mm Hg.

Bernice continues to use relaxation and imagery along with a modified low-salt diet and Aldactone (spironolactone) twice a week. Her blood pressure has been maintained at 150/90 mm Hg for three years.

Bernice's experience showed the staff that relaxation and imagery were a viable intervention. We also learned that no matter how ill a patient might be, it is important to maintain the individual's sense of control over his or her life. That loss of control is often more frightening than the illness itself. Bernice was able to regain some control over her life and eliminate a potentially fatal hypertensive state by using hypnosis.

Case Example: Longterm Patient

Steven, a 50-year-old scientist, came to me specifically for hypnosis because of labile hypertension and preventricular beats. His blood pressure had been normal until five years earlier, when he was hospitalized for a suspected kidney infection and his blood pressure reached 180/100 mm Hg. He was under the regular care of a private physician and had his blood pressure checked often by an allergist who administered shots every two weeks. He had been treated with diuretics and Inderal (propranolol, 25 mg b.i.d.) but was very motivated to find a nonchemical means of controlling his blood pressure. He was aware that stress seemed to aggravate his problem. Although he was a theoretical scientist and mathematician, he had a strong belief that the mind could control bodily functions and he practiced meditation regularly. He was not interested in psychotherapy, stating that he had many friends who were psychiatrists and that he had no particular problems in living except for circulatory ones. For the past year, his concern over his health had increased and he had begun to jog regularly and to watch his diet.

The hospital experience had created anxiety. Steven worried about what could be wrong with such a major organ as his heart and became preoccupied with the results of his tests. He was tense when his blood pressure was taken and gradually became extremely anxious with any stimulus related to this test, even the sound of the blood pressure machine being rolled down the hall. Because of his anxiety, when he visited the doctor his blood pressure was higher than it was at his allergist, where he did not feel so stressed.

Steven was one of two children raised in a traditional Jewish urban family. He described his mother as "crazy" and said that as she aged her behavior became increasingly bizarre. His younger sister was also a scientist and lived upstairs with her family. He was close to her and enjoyed their scientific conversations and sharing experiences between their families. Initially, he described her as ill with "some sort of immune disease" requiring him to donate blood for packed cell transfusions on a regular basis. When queried more about her illness, he denied it was particularly serious. He described himself as a bit "eccentric," a "flamboyant" teacher and non-neurotic, as happily married and the father of two lovely adolescent daughters. He denied a fear of death but admitted to not being "ready to go" and wanting to live a happy life. He had become more conscious of aging in the last year and was aware that his two daughters would soon be leaving home.

In investigating the meaning of Steven's chief complaint—hypertension and irregular heart rate—little information could be obtained and resistance was high. He did relate some instances he felt might be related. He stated that in high school, he had been so bright that he was accelerated. In college, as a result, he was younger than his peers and felt at times inadequate and insecure. He remembered a class that was both especially boring and particularly difficult. It was hard to stay awake. He discovered that by placing his fingers on his wrist, he could alter his pulse rate and remain alert. He was particularly adept at raising the rate. He also recalled flunking the physical for navigator's school in the Air Force because of an elevated pulse rate. He ended up a "second class" radio control operator and associated his "flunking the physical" to high anxiety.

During the initial interview, he denied any particular stress. Since he was an independent consultant, work was sporadic and therefore financially unpredictable. He also admitted to occasionally being aggravated and angry with his daughters. We discussed how anxiety and stress could influence blood pressure and PVCs. I also explained how relaxation and imagery procedures countered the effects of stress. These techniques, I said, could help him gain more control over his inner process. We discussed research in the field, and I explained that he would need to practice the techniques at home. He was encouraged to become more aware of when he was feeling stressed and anxious and to also be aware of what promoted relaxation and comfort. He was enthusiastic and willing to practice at home and to undertake other health-related activities that would aid in ameliorating his condition. His goal (not mine) was to become free of the beta-blocking medication.

I asked the patient what kind of imagery was relaxing to him. He described a place where he and his family went in the summer. It had a small house, trees, hills, and a stream. He also liked to run along a special road early in the morning. He enjoyed running and felt it put him into an exhilarating altered state. In this state, he felt his body worked well, he was relaxed and coordinated, and the physical exertion was easy and smooth.

I discussed hypnosis and answered his questions about it. I asked if he wanted to lay down or sit up; he chose to sit. I chose progressive relaxation and recreated the image he described. I suggested a sense of wholeness and health and that as he relaxed, exercised, and learned more about his inner processes, he would obtain his goal. The specific goal was left vague purposefully as an indirect suggestion, so that both consciously and unconsciously he would embellish his objective of managing blood pressure and heart rhythm if he chose to do so. I also told him that he could enter this nice state of relaxation and reverie whenever he wanted, and that the more he practiced the more adept he would become. I suggested that he could remember this state during times of stress and recreate it. I frequently told him that just as he was able to raise his pulse so many years ago, so would he be able to lower and regulate it *now* (an Ericksonian embedded command).

The process of treatment occured over a year, during which many issues were explored and numerous imagery and relaxation techniques taught. At each session, some discussion was related to how his life was going and if he was encountering stress. Over time the patient began to trust me and a more psychotherapeutic approach was utilized in conjunction with the imagery and relaxation techniques. Behavioral rehearsal, imagery techniques related to his heart, ego-building techniques, inner advisors, and self-regulating suggestions were all employed. He practiced the exercises at home, watched his diet, meditated, and jogged regularly. He also followed his physician's instructions, which were to take his medication "as needed." Very shortly after beginning treatment, he began reducing the beta-blocking medication and soon discontinued it entirely. His blood pressure was taken by his allergist and was found to be within normal limits. He seldom experienced PVCs.

After six weeks of treatment, Steven's sister died unexpectedly. This precipitated a major change in his therapy and provided an opportunity to discuss feelings within the context of his loss. He learned that she had had terminal leukemia, but had only told her husband of the seriousness of her illness. As we discussed her death, he described his feelings of shock and sadness. He was tearful but controlled. He stated he would miss her very much and that now whenever he practiced his relaxation, her face popped into his mind and the tears "streamed" down his face. This provided an opportunity to discuss normal grief, its symptoms, and how long it might last. I also stressed the potential healing value of seeing her image. He was encouraged to let himself feel and express it as best he could. We talked about men crying and how embarrassing it was for him. He reminisced about their life together growing up. Later in his treatment, probably as a result of these sessions, he was able to talk about his sadness over his older daughter's leaving home for college and how much he would miss her. He talked openly about the anger he felt about his sister's death and his daughter's leaving, as well as other aggravating experiences he was encountering. He began to discuss his own aging and other issues related to separation. In evaluating the treatment at termination, he stated that these sessions were especially useful as he had learned not to fear his feelings but to experience them as fully as possible. Most likely this aspect of the therapy helped him manage the stresses of living more effectively and hence influenced his ability to maintain a normal blood pressure, and eliminate his PVCs.

Many imagery techniques were employed during this process, some of which are described below.

Body Imagery Related to the Heart

Two images chosen by the patient were utilized to help Steven self-regulate his circulatory system.

E.T. (the little outer space creature from the 1982 film of the same name) had a regular, pulsating, warm glow that emanated from his chest, and this warmth was healing when extended out through his long distorted finger. The glow, in the movie, symbolized E.T.'s love and life. (Imagery that is enjoyed by the patient is the most likely to be successful.) The heart-warming image of E.T.'s glowing chest seemed a natural for Steven's problem. While in a relaxed trance state, he focused attention first on his hands. I used his hands because they are more sensitive than the chest. I then suggested the blood flow could increase and his hands become warmer and warmer. Ideomotor signaling was utilized so he could let me know when his hands were warm. Then he was asked to remember E.T. and the warm glow that emanated from his chest. I asked him to let the warmth in his hands transfer, if he wanted, to his chest. This was a complex series of events which linked the experience of warmth in the hands, a visual image of E.T., and a subsequent permissive suggestion to experience warmth in the chest. Taking the process in a step-by-step manner, and with practice, Steven was able to quickly experience his hands warming and his chest "glowing."

The second image was of a maintenance crew that cleaned and maintained Steven's blood vessels. I utilized self-disclosure as well as a discussion of research to introduce this image. I explained that when I had a sore throat or felt I was catching a "bug," I relaxed and imagined a maintenance crew with a very tough boss who directed his crew to attack the "bad germs and clean them out." I also described the Simmontons' imagery of valiant white knights killing evil cells in cancer patients. He imagined his circulatory system as having a series of strong maintenance men cleaning and taking care of his circulatory system. He enjoyed doing both exercises.

Behavioral Rehearsal and Biofeedback

Because Steven felt the elevated blood pressure occurred in association with the doctor's office, we decided to utilize a recreation of that experience. This resembled behavioral desensitization and behavioral rehearsal. In the relaxed trance state, he was encouraged to imagine going to his doctor's office, waiting for his appointment, entering the examining room, seeing the sphygmomanometer, having the cuff placed on his arm, and finally the reading done. He was gradually able to decrease his anxiety in the fantasized state. On several occasions, I took his pulse while he was doing the exercise and was able to feed back to him how he was doing. We also used this feedback technique to help him monitor and self-regulate the speed and rhythm of his heart.

Inner Advisor and Ego-Building Techniques

Throughout therapy, Steven was given positive suggestions that self-regulation, stress management, and good health could be his. I encouraged him to think of his body and mind as healthy; what he was doing to maintain health would pay off in normal blood pressure and heart rate. I pointed out his successes and told him often that his diligent practice, enthusiasm, and willingness to discuss his feelings would help him as a total person.

On several occasions, he expressed concern about his weight, and the treatment diverged into strategies for weight control. While he was not especially overweight, he worried that his periodic overeating could lead to obesity and malignant hypertension. I used several techniques for this, including ego-building, images of healthy food, and the use of the inner advisor (see Chapter 5). Steven imagined his inner advisor as a deer, but not just any deer; he was the mythical Lord of the deer whose function was to make sure that deer meat was not wasted. Steven had been a child during the Great Depression and remembered his family's emphasis on not wasting food. I pointed out to him how he now was misusing food by overeating; excess food was converted into useless fat (wasted). The deer spoke to him, without moving his mouth, in a very deep, stern wise voice, telling him not to waste food. He found this a valuable asset in both controlling his eating and in solving other problems as they occurred.

The imagery used with Steven developed over time and was used in conjunction with relaxation and both direct and indirect suggestions for change and control. While an attempt was made to determine more complex psychological meaning to his problem, what seemed to work best was the imagery developed from *both* our experiences. As he was a scientist and valued his independence, I purposefully chose an experimental approach—the two of us evaluating different approaches.

In follow-up I learned that Steven continued to maintain normal blood pressure and his routine of exercise and meditation using the images developed in therapy. He explained that he was still anxious when anticipating a physical in which his blood pressure would have to be taken, and that he sometimes took Inderal (propranolol) in such instances, as well as occasionally when he was unduly stresssed or had had a flu. However, he had not experienced any PVCs nor had any indication that his blood pressure was elevated.

SUMMARY

Hypnosis and hypnotic techniques can be a useful adjunct to the medical management of hypertension and other cardiovascular problems. Medical evaluation and monitoring are essential to prevent the progression of the disease. Nurses will usually work with these patients in conjunction with a physician. Both direct and indirect suggestive techniques, relaxation, imagery, and long- and short-term management are potential treatment modalities. These techniques augment not only medical management but also stress reduction, diet, and exercise, which are so important in managment of hypertension and cardiovascular disease. Utilization of relaxation and imagery can also be useful in group treatment with hypertensive patients.

REFERENCES

Alexander, F., French, T.M., & Pollock, G.H. (1968). *Psychosomatic specificity*. Chicago: University of Chicago Press.

Benson, H., Shapiro, D., Tursky, B., et al. (1971). Decreased systolic blood pressure through operant conditioning techniques. *Science, 173*, 740.

Benson, H. (1977). Systemic hypertension and relaxation response. *New England Journal of Medicine, 296*, 1152.

Brown, B. (1977). *Stress and the art of biofeedback*. New York: Bantam Books.

Case, D.B., Fogel, D.H., & Pollack, A.A. (1980). Intrahypnotic and longterm effects of self-hypnosis on blood pressure in mild hypertension. *International Journal of Clinical and Experimental Hypnosis, 28*, 27.

D'Atri, D.A., & Ostfeld, A.M. (1975). Crowding: Its effects on the elevation of blood pressure in a prison setting. *Preventative Medicine, 4*, 550–556.

Deabler, H.L., Fidel, E., Dillenkoffer, R.L., et al. (1973). The use of relaxation and hypnosis in lowering high blood pressure. *American Journal of Clinical Hypnosis, 16*, 75.

Editor's note (1980). *Behavioral Medicine, 7*, 4.

Falkner, B., Onesti, G., & Hamstra, B. (1981). Stress response characteristics of adolescents with high genetic risks for essential hypertension: A five-year follow-up. *Clinical and Experimental Hypertension, 3*, 583–591.

Friedman, H., & Taub, H. (1978). A six month follow-up of the use of hypnosis and biofeedback procedures in essential hypertension. *American Journal of Clinical Hypnosis, 20*, 184.

Grahm, J.D. (1945). High blood pressure with battle. *Lancet, 1*, 239.

Guyton, A.C. (1980). *Arterial pressure and hypertension*. Philadelphia: W.B. Saunders.

Harburg, E., Blakelock, E., & Roger, P. (1979). Resentful and reflective coping with arbitrary authority and blood pressure. *Detroit Psychosomatic Medicine, 41*, 189–202.

Harrell, J. (1980). Psychological factors and hypertension: A status report. *Psychology Bulletin, 87*, 482–501.

Henry, J.P., & Cassel, J.C. (1969). Psychosocial factors in essential hypertension: Recent epidemiological and animal experimental evidence. *American Journal of Epidemiology, 90*, 171.

Kasl, S.V., & Cobb, S. (1970). Blood pressure changes in men undergoing job loss: A preliminary report. *Psychosomatic Medicine, 32*, 19.

Lane, A., & Ruskin, A. (1950). A note on the failure of hypnosis in essential hypertension. *Texas Republic Biological Medicine, 8*, 66.

May, J., & Johnson, H. (1973). Physiological activity to internally-elicited arousal and inhibitory thoughts. *Journal of Abnormal Psychology, 82*, 239–245.

Reiser, M.F., Brust, A.A., & Fures, E.F. (1951). Life situations, emotions and the course of patients with arterial hypertension. *Psychosomatic Medicine, 13*, 133.

Sheikh, A.A., Richardson, P., and Moleski, L.M. Psychosomatics and mental imagery: A brief review, in A.A. Sheikh and J.T. Shaffer (Eds.) *The potential of fantasy and imagination*. New York: Brandon House, 1979.

Speigel, H. (1973). *Manual for hypnotic induction profile: eye-roll levitation method*, rev. ed. New York: Soni Medica.

Taylor, C.B., & Fortman, S.P. (1983). Essential hypertension. *Psychosomatics, 24,* 443–447.

Wadden, T.A., & de la Torre, C.S. (1980). Relaxation therapy as adjunct treatment for hypertension, *Journal of Family Practice, 11,* 901–908.

Weiner, H. (1977). *The psychobiology of human illness,* New York: Elsevier.

Hypnotic Techniques with Dying Patients and Those Who Fear Death

By Rothlyn P. Zahourek*

RELEVANT CONCEPTUAL FRAMEWORKS

Hypnotic techniques have several applications with terminally ill patients or with those who are fearful of dying.* Because the definition of "dying" is not always easy, dying patients and those fearful of dying will be grouped together. The problems of the severely ill or injured patient likewise fit into this category. Their problems and concerns are similar and the hypnotic interventions are often interchangeable, although the therapeutic process may differ markedly. These similar concerns include pain, disrupted body image, fear, isolation, hopelessness, and a sense of lost control. For the patient who is actually terminal, medical management can only arrest the course of the disease for a short period of time, and death is expected in the near rather than distant future. These patients have the additional burden (and some feel privilege) of saying goodbye to life and loved ones and tying up the loose ends of their lives. Grieving is a natural although painful part of this process for both the patient and for those associated with him or her.

Relaxation, guided imagery, distraction, and pain relief often help the terminally ill complete their lives with dignity and comfort. Wallace LaBaw (1969) described his work with two terminally ill patients, demonstrating that through hypnosis these patients remained comfortable, optimistic, and highly functional even though physically debilitated.

Crasilneck and Hall (1975) outlined several purposes for hypnosis with

---

*Case example "Jimmy" supplied by Marcia Fishman.
*See Chapter 10 for additional information on the dying child.

cancer patients and suggested that not all patients are candidates. Those who
(1) want to avoid medications that cloud their awareness, (2) wish to control
pain without narcotics, (3) wish to delay cachexia by maintaining adequate food
intake, and (4) want to end their lives as alert and comfortable as possible are
ideal candidates. Hypnosis relieves pain, reduces the anxiety and discomfort of
tests and treatments, helps maintain appetite, decreases side effects from chemotherapy and radiation, and promotes an active, relatively hopeful emotional
state (LaBaw, 1975; Chong, 1968). Two important advantages of hypnosis are
mentioned by Crasilneck and Hall (1975). First, hypnosis focuses the patient's
attention on the most immediate problem and involves a caregiver who provides a technique to cope with that particular problem. This reassures the
patient that he or she will not be abandoned and that their immediate needs
will be addressed. Secondly, patients can be passively at ease and the object of
attention by a caring adult without loosing self-esteem.

Hypnosis helps deal with the fears of the dying experience itself. Sheikh
(1983, 1979) described visiting one's own death in the imagination. He felt that
fear of the unknown is diminished and a new sense of meaning in life is accomplished when one encounters what death might actually be like. "Purposeful
life is possible only through an unflinching acceptance of death as an integral
constituent of life; confronting death draws one to the threshold of life
. . . paradoxically (this) often leads to 'life giving experiences'" (Sheikh & Jor-
dan, 1983, p. 412).

Bruce Greyson (1983) reviewed several studies of near-death experiences.
He stated that near-death experiences (actual rather than imaginary) foster
value transformation and decrease suicidal ideation in patients who become
depressed, and he speculated that this decrease may be due to a decathexis of
past personal failures.

Because of the impact of near-death (real or imagined) experiences on
one's value system, an imagery exercise is useful in education of caregivers.
Several years ago Carol Alexander conducted a dramatic role play exercise in a
death and dying workshop. I will never forget sitting on the floor in pairs, back
to back in a darkened room as she explained, "You have just been in an earth-
quake, and the building you were in has caved in. You are with one other
person but you can't see that person, only talk with them. You know you have
been severely injured and you are experiencing symptoms of shock. You're cold
and somewhat lightheaded. Your partner is likewise seriously injured. You
know if help does not come soon that you will die." We were instructed to tell
our partner any last messages we had for loved ones, to write our epitaph, and
to write down the name of any person or situation we had unresolved feelings
about. We had a chance to finish anything that was left undone and to write
messages. We were then told that our partner had become quiet and had
probably died. We were alone in the dark and growing weaker ourselves. We
were encouraged to think quietly about what our lives had meant. This moving

exercise precipitates intense feelings and sometimes tears. It, however, sensitizes the nurse to what the dying patient experiences.*

Similarly, significant others can be helped to anticipate the death and dying experience through imagery and hypnotic techniques. In addition, a new involvement may develop as the significant other aids the patient in pain management or in helping the patient obtain a sense of ease and well-being. Having something helpful to do enables them to feel useful and subsequently decreases their anxiety and sense of hopelessness and helplessness.

It would seem an oversight to discuss the terminal patient and the use of imagery and not to describe the work of the Simmontons (Simmonton & Simmonton, 1975). Their work has been especially important as it focuses on the integration of mind, body, and spirit to slow the process of, and increase the recovery rate from, cancer. In recent years their work has received a great deal of publicity. They report that many people treated with their approach, which combines medical and surgical management, psychotherapy, family involvement, and guided, healing imagery, have experienced remission, and some even cure. Their work has stimulated numerous popular books on self-healing (Cousins, 1976; Simmonton & Simmonton, 1979). While the Simmontons have documented numerous successful cases, the inconsistent results of others using their techniques have perpetuated scientific skepticism. Similarly, the link between a particular personality type and stress has not been demonstrated to be connected to the development of cancer. For these reasons, and probably also because of resistance to belief in mind–body connections, widespread acceptance has not been sufficient so that their approaches have not become part of the standard care plan for cancer patients. Nonetheless many health care workers use their approach, believing that positive attitudes, dealing with conflict, and visualizing body processes work for many individuals and provide a better prognosis. We know relaxation reduces tension and opens constricted blood vessels, thereby improving circulation and potential healing to an affected part. Likewise we know that the immune system is influenced by stress, anxiety, and depression. Positive self-image, hope, and comfort are affective states in which most individuals are likely to cooperate with treatment recommendations. For all these reasons the Simmontons' approach certainly should be considered with both cancer and other seriously ill patients (an interesting discussion of their work occurs by Maggie Scarf in *Psychology Today*, Sept., 1980).

Because many publications are currently promoting these ideas, it is well for the nurse to be cognizant that the general population may be both receptive to these techniques and harboring unrealistic hopes for cure. A delicate balance exists between a realistic, positive attitude and an overzealous approach that

---

*Similar exercises can be found in *The dying patient: Learning processes for interaction*, by Charlotte Epstein. Reston, VA: Reston Publishing, 1975.

may be detrimental or cause the patient to avoid potentially useful traditional medical management. However, many who utilize these techniques have witnessed often surprising and very positive results. Cautions, care, and intelligent case assessment are encouraged, as well as a positive attitude that results can promote comfort and better quality of life. This is different from promising a miracle cure.

Health care workers should stay current with new research on the relationship of stress to health and stress to cancer. We know now that the relationship between stress and disease is not a simplistic one. Individual responses to similar stressors vary greatly, and some (actually unknown) quantity of stress mobilizes the natural defenses and is necessary for the triggering of the immune system. Likewise, mental attitudes do not always affect prognosis in a linear fashion. A recent news article (*Psychology Today,* 1983) reported a preliminary study by Sandra Levy at the National Cancer Institute, finding that women with early-stage breast cancer who were depressed had a poor prognosis for survival. On the other hand, women who had recurrent breast cancer and had little chance of survival but who reported depression, anxiety, hostility, and fatigue were more likely to survive a year than women with "more positive attitudes."

No accurate predictors exist at present for who with a particular mental attitude will do well physiologically at a particular stage of illness and who will not. Nevertheless, it is generally believed that a positive attitude and a positive prognosis seem generally related, whether the patient is terminal or not. Comfort and a sense of meaning similarly remain priorities for patient and family.

Hypnotic techniques provide for the development of a helping relationship with the patient who feels alone and isolated. Commonly in the dying process both patient and loved ones withdraw emotional attachments because they think it will ease the pain of saying goodbye. For the dying, this includes numerous people and life itself. Withdrawal may be extreme but is protective and adaptive. Likewise family, friends, and even caregivers withdraw from the dying out of helplessness, grief and difficulties with separation. Other times the patient's pain, if unmanaged, produces guilt and such discomfort in the staff and loved ones that, once again, the dying patient is avoided. For the patient and those involved, avoidance is an attempt at "out of sight out of mind," but the less conscious mental process of grieving continues, often surfacing to awareness in nightmares, fantasy, and dreams. Many mourners explain that they feel "fine" (don't think about their sadness and loss) while awake and busy with usual activities. However, when they lie down and close their eyes to sleep, they are flooded with mental pictures, imagined sounds, sensations, and associated feelings. Hospital sights, noises, and smells are vividly re-experienced or projected. Often if the person has had no previous close association with dying, the images are doubly frightening or unrealistic.

When death is unexpected, disbelief may be problematic. Whether death is expected or sudden, letting go is painful. Allowing loved ones to care for the dying person, and after death, to see the body for as long as desired allows not only for needed goodbyes but also for a "mental picture" of that person as dying, and then as dead, to be firmly implanted so that acceptance can gradually occur. Some will wish to remember the person as he or she was and will avoid seeing the dead body. This however may delay acceptance and block grief resolution, leaving possible distorted images and fantasies. Related to this need for an accurate mental picture are the search for bodies after a disaster, and "viewings" associated with funerals.

Imagery is an essential aspect of the grief process. Early in grief the image of the lost person is idealized; later anger over the loss may devalue the memory. Resolution occurs when the images become more balanced.

Within this context, hypnotic techniques offer those working with the dying, and the grieving significant others, opportunities to reassure people that their fantasies are a normal part of grieving and to help them find positive distractions if these images become too intense. Guided fantasy can program thinking and provide mental relief.

These techniques require active involvement of both the patient and the caregiver. Since the patient tends to be comforted, caregivers feel a sense of usefulness and relief. The patient is less isolated because caregivers experience success and are more capable of remaining involved with those most draining of patients.

In addition to patients who are actually dying, nurses encounter patients who fear death or who develop ideas that they have a terminal illness when in fact they do not. These patients can be difficult and may need additional psychotherapy.

APPROACHES WITH PATIENTS WHO ARE PREOCCUPIED WITH UNREALISTIC FEARS OF ILLNESS AND DEATH

Patients in numerous health care settings have medical problems and psychosomatic symptoms, and may develop unrealistic attitudes about their health. Dynamically these symptoms can portray unresolved conflicts and needs that cannot be expressed any other way.

Case #1: Fear of Death with Surgery

A long term psychotherapy patient, Penny, discovered she had a pelvic mass which required surgery. While told the likelihood of malignancy was minimal, she was convinced it was metastasized cancer. If the rapidly growing mass was left unattended it would probably rupture and cause peritonitis, but for several weeks Penny refused surgery, feeling she did not want to add pain to

---

*See also Chapter 7. The description of "Rose" demonstrates hypnosis with a dying patient who is in crisis because of intense pain.

what would be only a little more time to live. Her refusal precipitated power struggles with her physician, her friends, and me. She felt no one really cared what she wanted. Clearly she was on a self-destructive path. Finally, after a positive conversation with her physician and several therapy sessions exploring her motivations and anger at authority figures, she decided to have the operation. The fear of dying, however, continued.

We began relaxation exercises to help with the anxiety. She was receptive and practiced at home. Anxiety about the outcome, however, continued and she could not control thoughts that she would die either during the surgery or soon after. A week before the scheduled surgery, we did a visualization exercise, hoping to encourage thoughts of a positive outcome. After a relaxation procedure, I asked Penny to imagine herself being prepped and readied for the surgery.

"See yourself being wheeled to the operating room and positioned on the table. Remember your nice relaxation exercises. You are breathing regularly and feeling comfortable. Allow yourself to relax even more as the anesthesiologist begins the anesthesia." She looked more anxious. "See yourself on the table and notice that the procedure is going well. Everything is going much better than you expected." She looked even more anxious and tense; her breathing was rapid and her forehead deeply furrowed. Her body was nearly rigid. "Relax and see that the procedure is going well." She still looked very uncomfortable. I finally said, "It appears that you are very uncomfortable and that you either have pain or things are not going as well as you had hoped. Try and see that things are going better now and the outcome will be better." She still looked just as miserable and upset. With her eyes closed she related a very frightening experience; she had had a cardiac arrest on the table and no one could do anything to help and revive her. She saw herself being wrapped in a shroud and taken from the operating room to the morgue. People were very matter of fact. It was cold; she was put on a slab and then in the morgue drawer. I told her then that we were going to change the scene completely. "Go to that favorite place you enjoy so much. Go away from that previous experience and relax very deeply and comfortably." Now she looked relaxed, peaceful, rested, and comfortable. Soon after I asked her to open her eyes so we could talk about what she experienced. She now looked pale, shaken, and sad. The experience frightened her very much. She had never carried her fantasies specifically and vividly to their conclusion—her death. Characteristically, she became withdrawn and angry in the session, seeming unable to express herself verbally.

I too was shaken by her spontaneous visualization and was even more concerned about the potential outcome of the surgery. I remembered that patients who strongly believed they would die in surgery often did. I was also disheartened she had not been able to interrupt the negative image to one of a positive outcome even in the comfortable relaxed state. I noted she was able to go in her imagination to a favorite vacation spot and feel good. I was invested in her being able in some way to experience the upcoming surgery in a positive way; I felt the pressure of time, as the surgery was scheduled for a few days hence.

After consultation with a colleague, I learned that Penny's death fantasy was probably part of her angry need to both control and to get back at authoritarian people, particularly her parents. I confronted this power struggle and directly told her I thought some of the need to die was a desire for revenge at supposedly powerful people who let her down. I mentioned her mother's desertion of her when she was an ill child, my powerlessness to take adversity away, and incidents of the physician's insensitivity as all grounds for her to punish us. The stakes, however, were very high. She replied that this was probably an accurate interpretation. She also mentioned feeling somewhat better and that she was willing to continue the relaxation and imagery exercises. I noted that in the past when using imagery she had visualized the worst possible consequences, reacted to them, and let them go, and then envisioned a positive outcome. I emphasized that during the previous session, she was able to move from a fearful, negative and indeed "dead" state to one of relaxation and comfort on her favorite beach. I hypothesized that if she could do it then, she could also do it when she experienced negative thoughts. I encouraged her to remember this when she practiced and that, after all, she had suffered for the last six months over this upcoming surgery and she deserved some pleasure (indirect suggestion that she can change). She agreed. I was not scheduled to see her again until the night before surgery. I hoped the indirect suggestions would take hold, that she would be able to modify the experience, and that overall she had good results from imagining the absolute worst. I knew she would call if having difficulty; I did not hear from her.

The night before surgery, she looked perky, sitting in her hospital bed in a new nightgown. Several people dropped by to see her; she was receptive and cheerful. She felt hopeful about the surgery and realized that she needed to carry her fantasy to its most dreaded conclusion in order to feel relief. She had been practicing relaxation using a "worry stone" which she proudly showed me, stating it was going to the operating room with her.

The surgery went without mishap, she recovered without complication, and both of us were greatly relieved.

Discussion

This hospitalization and surgery rekindled in Penny the feelings associated with a prior traumatic hospitalization as well as experiences she had during childhood illnesses. Hypnotic techniques provided her with a chance to experience nonverbally what she most feared. For her this was especially appropriate since throughout therapy she had experienced difficulty putting feelings into words. Carrying her fantasy to the extreme allowed for an intense emotional reaction and catharsis. Subsequently, she was more rationally able to plan a hopeful course of action. Noteworthy is that even though I tried to create a positive image regarding the surgery, she was intent on carrying the fantasy to a

negative conclusion. Confronting her anger at parents and other authority figures, in addition to the powerful reaction to the imagery exercise, moved her
quickly toward restructured thinking and more optimistic feelings. One doesn't
know if she would have accomplished this without the imagery. My sense is she
might not have in time for the surgery, since she was nonverbal and minimally
psychologically minded.

HYPNOTIC APPROACHES WITH DYING PATIENTS

Many patients consciously ready themselves for death. Preparations for
their death can be rather extensive, and it may seem incredible how much
control they exert over the last "season" of their lives. Nurses have a unique
contribution to make in their preparations.

The Power of Imagery with a Dying Child*

I am not a pediatric nurse. Dealing with seriously ill children leaves me
emotionally and physically drained. I tell you this to give you some idea of what
it was like to see Jimmy as a client.

I was packing for a working vacation when I received a call from an extremely distraught father asking me to see his 7-year-old son who was dying of
leukemia. I tried to explain that I did not handle children. The father insisted I
try. Jimmy was at home because it was what he wanted and his parents and
physician felt best for him. Jimmy was at a point where he was in terrible pain
and could not keep even minimal food or liquids down. Worse still was Jimmy's
continuous fight against sleep, because if he closed his eyes he was afraid he
would die. Not medication, nor being home, nor loving parents were able to
console Jimmy or stop his pain. His physician suggested hypnosis and steered
the parents to me.

I realized this would be a one-time attempt. I could not say no.

Jimmy was emaciated and dehydrated, with a swollen belly and painful
joints. His eyes were sunken, his skin yellow, and he was tachypneic. He was in
a tight fetal position with fists tightly clenched. When I first laid eyes on him I
physically withdrew from him and verbally expressed my dismay—not the best
way to establish rapport with a child. Jimmy was very aware of my presence and
reaction. There was no retreat. I looked at this wide-eyed child and said, "I'm
sorry, Jimmy, I didn't realize how sick you really are." He quickly acknowledged my explanation with a nod of his head.

I went on to explain who I was and that I was there to help him feel much
better. Did he know how to pretend? Again a nod. I asked him to close his

---

*This story is retold by permission from the Foundation of Thanatology, 722 W. 168th St.,
New York, NY where it has been published in their archives.

eyes. Could he see a picture of a boat in his head? A nod. His favorite toy? A nod. His Mommy and Daddy? A nod. Open your eyes Jimmy. He did. "Jimmy, can you tell me what it's like to be sick?" He said, "It's cold, dark, lonely, and hurts a lot. I'm afraid. I'm very thirsty but if I drink anything I start to throw up and then I hurt more. I can't play anymore. I miss my friends and school." Jimmy then showed me a picture he had drawn. It was on legal-sized paper, totally colored in heavy black crayon, except for one small square in the lower right-hand corner, where a simple picture of a stick figure in fetal position on a bed was drawn.

I said, "Jimmy, tell me where you would like to sit when we play 'let's pretend.'" He chose his father's reclining chair, with a pillow behind his back so he could sit upright. His father carried him into the den and settled Jimmy into the chair. I assured Jimmy that Mommy and Daddy were going to be in the room and we would not do anything to make him hurt more.

At this time, I asked Jimmy to close his eyes and to "slowly breathe in and out." Even though his breathing rate was very rapid, I maintained a slow, calm, rhythm and tone. After several minutes, when I saw his breathing begin to slow down a bit, I said, "Jimmy, can you breathe in through your nose and out through your mouth?" His eyes opened wide. "I don't know what you mean. Show me." Once I demonstrated, Jimmy said, "I can do that." He gave a return demonstration. Then I asked him to do it with his eyes closed. He promptly closed his eyes and proceeded to breathe evenly and calmly. Jimmy's breathing had markedly slowed down, maintaining the rhythm I set. His facial expression began to show a decrease in tension, but his arms and legs were still tightly flexed and his fists clenched. I wanted to see if he would continue to follow my directions. I asked him to breathe faster, and I speeded up the rhythm.

"Very good, Jimmy. Notice how much better you're beginning to feel. Now let's slow down your breathing. Nice and easy. In, out, in, out. You're doing wonderful. You're feeling so much better. Jimmy, can you feel your arms and legs getting looser and looser?" I continued reinforcing his feeling better and better and his legs and arms getting more relaxed and looser. After three or four minutes, he straightened his legs and let his arms rest at his sides. "Jimmy, can you tell me about your favorite toy?" With a great big smile, he said, "Dog." (Jimmy cuddled the toy as if he were really holding it.) "He's big, brown, soft, and warm and he doesn't hurt." In actuality, "Dog" was in the room on the couch, a ragged, nondescript, stuffed toy.

I asked, "How would you like to take Dog and go to the park with me?" Shaking his head yes, he put out his hand while still clutching Dog.

I said, "You're going to have to show me the way because I don't know how to get to the park."

As we walked down the street, he told me who lived in the different houses. He even gave me the name of the big dog on the corner. Jimmy assured me the dog didn't bite.

Jimmy: Oh, boy! I see the swings.

Marcia: Would you like to get on the swings? (Nodding yes, Jimmy handed Dog to me.)

Marcia: Would you like me to push you?

Jimmy: No, I can do it myself.

Marcia: Very good. You are feeling stronger. Jimmy, you are going higher and higher. The higher you go the better and stronger you feel.

I let Jimmy play in the playground for about ten minutes. We watched his little body relax more and more.

Marcia: Look how high you're going. You look much better. Do you feel better?

Jimmy: I don't hurt so much now.

Marcia: Jimmy, it's time to leave the park now. We have another place to go and visit. I gave Jimmy time to slow down and get off the swing. Once off the swing, he asked for Dog back and again took my hand.

I said, "Now we're going to visit a different place. We're going to visit where death is and see what it's like." Jimmy immediately withdrew his hand and again rolled into a tight fetal position. I said, "Jimmy, remember this is just 'Let's pretend.' I promised nothing can hurt you. Mommy and Daddy are here. I am here and nothing will hurt you." Jimmy relaxed a bit, took my hand and again straightened out in the chair.

Marcia: Jimmy, tell me what death looks like.

Jimmy: I'm scared.

Marcia: Don't be frightened, it's only "Let's pretend.' (Pause) "Can you tell me what death is like?"

Jimmy: It's very black and cold. I'm all alone and scared, and it makes me hurt.

I realized Jimmy's description of death was exactly the same as his earlier picture of what it was like to be very ill. I said, "Jimmy, I know what's wrong now. You are not seeing death. You are seeing what it was like being sick all this time. You're looking in the wrong place. Turn your head to the left. (He did.) Do you see the beautiful light? (He nodded yes.) Let's you and I go see where the light is coming from. Remember, nothing will hurt you, so you can peek in and see how different death is from being sick." Jimmy held my hand tighter. In the other he clutched Dog. We walked through the dark and cold together.

Marcia: Are we there yet? (Jimmy nodded yes) Okay, now push the door open and tell me what you see?

Jimmy: (Suddenly excited) Grandpa! Grandpa is smiling and waving to me (Jimmy's mother and father were surprised at this description). And my goldfish, they're here too!

He also described the park and its playground, even the swings. Then I noticed a change in Jimmy's face.

Marcia: Jimmy, can you tell me what is wrong?

Jimmy: (Sadly) I don't see any other children here.

Marcia: (Knowing Jimmy liked school) "I'll bet they're in school."

This seemed to satisfy Jimmy. He became very serious. "When I die Grandpa is going to meet me. But if I die I'll leave Mommy and Daddy and my sister."

Jimmy's parents were on the edges of their seats. I motioned for them to stay there and tried to reassure them with quiet hand signals that all was okay. I felt it was something that could be handled. I said, "Yes, Jimmy, you are going to leave them. But remember, they are going to know you and Grandpa are happy together. Mommy and Daddy will know that you are well and don't hurt any more. You and Grandpa will be able to watch over your Mommy, Daddy, and little sister."

Jimmy appeared very relaxed and accepted my explanation with a simple "Yes." At this point, I felt very tired.

Marcia: I think it's time we go back home now.

Jimmy: Hold my hand when we pass through the dark.

Marcia: Now that we're almost home, I will soon slowly count to three. On three, you can open your eyes. When you open your eyes, you will feel much better. . . . I'll bet you're hungry and thirsty from all this playing and walking.

Jimmy: Yes. Can I visit these places again?

Marcia: Yes, Mommy and Daddy will know how to help you with "Let's pretend." Playing this helped you feel much better, didn't it?

Jimmy: Yes.

Marcia: (Slowly) One . . . two . . . three. . . . You may open your eyes.

Jimmy opened his eyes and smiled. "I liked that. Can I have some milk?" Mommy and Daddy and I were all quietly crying. There was a remarkable change in Jimmy. When he saw us, he put his hand on his hip and shook his head in dismay. "I don't know why you're crying. I feel much better." This made it even more difficult for me. My God, I thought, this child will never have a chance to learn that one can cry from happiness too.

Jimmy had his snack and went to sleep for the first time in several days. His mother, father and I sat together discussing what had been accomplished and how they could do the same. They were still shocked by Jimmy's having seen Grandpa. It was then I learned his beloved Grandpa had always lived with them. A little over a year before, Grandpa was suddenly rushed to the hospital by ambulance. The last time Jimmy saw his Grandpa was when the attendants carried him out of the house on a stretcher. Jimmy asked to visit Grandpa, but this was not allowed. Grandpa died in the hospital about a week later. Jimmy's parents told him of Grandpa's death. Jimmy did not ask questions. Mommy and Daddy did not think he would understand so they gave no explanation. Jimmy was not taken to the wake or funeral as his parents felt it would be too upsetting. Jimmy did not mention Grandpa again. Six months later, Jimmy was diagnosed with leukemia.

I left for my working vacation the following morning. When I returned two weeks later, his parents called to tell me Jimmy had passed away. His death had been at home and peaceful. Jimmy's parents used imagery over his last days to control much of the discomfort. Using imagery they took him to the park where he would go on the swings and seesaw, play with his friends and sister. This always reduced his pain and made him hungry and thirsty. Often, they did it before bedtime and gave the suggestion of his getting very tired. Jimmy was able to sleep more restfully. Whenever they did imagery, Jimmy and his parents would hold hands. Sometimes they let his little sister participate. The parents felt very positive about their experience. It gave them a way to help comfort their dying son, and brought the family closer together. The parents also found it decreased their own anxiety and made it easier for them to handle the stress they were feeling. Most importantly, Jimmy and his sister were again able to share time together, including several good sibling fights. When Jimmy had been in severe pain, dehydrated, and without sleep, he had become very frightening to his little sister. That had stopped once he felt better.

Jimmy asked to visit death several more times before his death. Though a little uncomfortable at first, his parents did not deny him. They always had to pass through the cold and black first. Once there, Jimmy would peek in. He always saw Grandpa waiting for him. Sometimes he would see other children playing. They were smiling and waiting for him to come soon.

The night he died, he asked to visit "Grandpa" (not death). When his mother said she would take him, Jimmy stated, "It's okay, we don't have to play 'Let's pretend' tonight." Jimmy died quietly in his sleep that night.

I have been in touch with the family several times since then. They are all doing well. For me it was difficult. I will never forget my first look into Jimmy's terrified eyes. But I will also never forget the change in Jimmy after our "Let's pretend."

This case example needs little summary, other than that it powerfully exemplifies the unique role a caregiver can play with the dying and their significant others. Hypnosis can augment that role.

> There are many similarities between . . . birth and death. In childhood the conscious mind slowly emerges from the oceanic feeling of immersion in unconsciousness.
>
> As death approaches, the conscious personality seems to be reemersed gradually in the unconscious. Both processes are facilitated by the presence of a caring person. (Crasilneck and Hall, 1975).

Working with the dying and those fearful of dying can be extremely taxing. It stimulates our own fears of dying and losing loved ones, and often we avoid these patients when they need us the most. Caregivers are encouraged, therefore, to visit their own imaginary deaths to have a fuller appreciation for both their patients and for their own lives.

REFERENCES

Chong, T.M. (1968). The use of hypnosis in management of patients who have cancer. *Singapore Medical Journal*, 9, 211–214.

Cousins, N. (1976). Anatomy of an illness. *New England Journal of Medicine*. 295, 1458–1463.

Crasilneck, H.B., & Hall, J.A. (1975). *Clinical hypnosis: Principles and applications.* New York: Grune & Stratton.

Diagnostic and statistical manual of mental disorders (ed. 3) (1981). Washington, D.C.: American Psychiatric Association.

Greyson, B. (1983). Near death experiences and personal values. *American Journal of Psychiatry, 140,* 5.

LaBaw, W.L., Helton, C., Tewell, K., & Eccles, D. (1975). Use of hypnosis by children with cancer. *American Journal of Clinical Hypnosis, 17,* 233–238.

LaBaw, W.L. (1969). Terminal hypnosis in lieu of terminal hospitalization: An effective alternative in fortunate cases. *Gerontology Clinic, 11,* 312–320.

Pelletier, K.R. (1977). *Mind as healer; Mind as slayer.* New York: Dell.

Psychology Today, 17, 11, Nov., 1983. (Report in Cross Talk section).

Scarf, M. (1980). Images that heal: A doubtful idea whose time has come. *Psychology Today, 14,* 32–46.

Sheikh, A.A. (Ed.) (1983). Imagery: Current theory, research and application. New York: John Wiley & Sons.

Sheikh, A.A., Twente, G.E., & Guerner, D. (1979). Death imagery: Therapeutic uses. In Sheikh, A.A., & Shaffer, J.T., (Eds.), *The potential of fantasy and imagination.* New York: Brandon House.

Simmonton, O.C., & Simmonton, S. (1975). Belief systems and management of the emotional aspects of malignancy. *Journal of Transpersonal Psychotherapy.* 7, 29–48.

Simmonton, O.C., & Simmonton, S. (1979). *Getting well again.* Los Angeles: Tarcher.

16

Hypnotic Techniques in Psychotherapy

Rothlyn P. Zahourek

THE LEGACY OF HYPNOSIS IN PSYCHOTHERAPY

Hypnosis has a special legacy and relevance for all psychotherapists as it played a crucial role in the development of Freudian theory and the practice of psychoanalysis. It was through hypnosis that Freud mapped the "royal road" to the unconscious. His early psychotherapy incorporated hypnosis and his patients reported fantasies and dreams while in a trance state. As a result of these experiences, Freud developed his theories of the unconscious and learned that childlike fantasies (primary process thinking) intruded into adult mental processes. According to Freud the well analyzed adult would overcome this and rely mainly on logical, secondary process thinking. While Freud later rejected hypnosis and adopted free association as a therapeutic technique, the modern analytic process resembles hypnosis. The patient, placed in a reclining position in an atmosphere of reduced stimuli, is encouraged to focus inward, to fantasize and to talk about whatever comes to mind; recall of early memories is encouraged. Although some analysts deny using hypnosis, many analytic patients probably enter a "trance state" spontaneously.

Early in the development of psychoanalysis Jung, a colleague of Freud's, disagreed with him over the importance of fantasy and the imagination. Jung believed in the 'adaptive, pleasurable or enriching quality of wishful imagery laden thinking' which Freud had 'downplayed in favor of directed, logical thought' (Singer and Pope, 1978 p. 5). This magical, primary process thinking which utilizes the creative and healing potential of the imagination is now not only the emphasis in Jungian psychotherapy but is also at the heart of therapy incorporating hypnosis or imagery processes (cognitive and behavioral therapies, biofeedback, neurolinguistic programming and Gestalt therapies, to name but a few).

These newer therapies played a role in the most recent revolution (1950–70) in psychiatry. This revolution restructured the care of patients in mental hospitals and encouraged shorter term more reality based therapies geared toward reaching a broader based population than traditional psychoanalysis. These therapies utilized techniques for reducing stress, natural noninvasive methods for symptom management or removal and techniques promoting cognitive, emotional and behavioral changes. Hypnotic approaches often utilized in these therapies aimed at reducing the length, and increasing the effectiveness of treatment. A revival of interest in hypnosis is causing new research and renewed interest in hypnosis in the context of psychotherapy.

Psychiatric nursing has a somewhat similar legacy. Traditionally, psychiatric nurses drew on major psychoanalytic, behavioral, and developmental theory. The emphasis in practice was and continues to be largely on the therapeutic relationship, behavioral management, understanding sociocultural influences, building self-esteem and coping capacities, and utilizing the interpersonal process therapeutically. An integrated (mind–body), multivariable understanding of people has influenced psychiatric nursing therapy.

In 1957 Hildegard Peplau described consciousness on a continuum and the importance of appreciating this continuum in nursing practice. She stressed that nurses must utilize their own experience, coupled with theory and observations, to understand behavior. The following quote illustrates ideas of therapists and theorists who are predominantly associated with hypnosis. She stated that the nurse must have "an understanding of the concepts of awareness and unawareness, attention and inattention, especially with regard to relations between feelings, thoughts and actions . . . to grasp the hidden meaning of symptoms and other forms of communication used by patients."

This sounds remarkably like present-day Rogerian (Martha) theory (1970), which has been so influential on nursing practice (see also Chapter 1). Both Peplau and Rogers described an approach that closely resembles hypnosis.

Generally it seems that psychiatric nurses have been unafraid to experiment with new ideas, to utilize current research findings, and to decide what works best with their particular client population. The breakthrough of nurses into community mental health, general hospital liaison and consultation, and private practice, as well as the availability of analytic and postgraduate psychotherapy training, have all contributed to and encouraged nurses' advanced study and subsequent expert practice as psychotherapists. Over the past 20 years psychiatric nurses have become increasingly independent, accountable, and innovative in a variety of practice situations.

THE USES OF HYPNOSIS IN PSYCHOTHERAPY
AND PSYCHIATRIC NURSING

The term *hypnotic techniques* is used to apply to the techniques of relaxation, suggestion and imagery. *Hypnosis* refers to formal induction of an altered state, with specific suggestions accompanying the induction. This chapter will provide clinical examples of both as they are used in clinical psychotherapy situations.

The beauty of hypnotic techniques is they can be utilized in many ways and integrated into most standard approaches with various kinds of patients: Inpatient unit nurses use positive suggestion unconsciously and routinely as they interact with both patients and staff. Relaxation groups are common now to help patients cope with stress and anxiety. Informal imagery exercises could easily be utilized in such instances as anticipating discharge and making future plans. Those in outpatient and private practice situations generally encounter healthier clients who might be more capable of using more complex techniques in short-term and long-term therapy. Those in general hospital consultation-liaison positions are in an ideal setting to implement hypnotic techniques. The nurse consultant is usually called to help with patients on whom the staff has given up; because the situation has become desperate, both staff and patient are willing to try "anything." Hypnosis often is appropriate, highly effective, and interesting and fun for staff and patients, providing a new context for a therapeutic relationship (Zahourek, 1982).

Whether or not a psychotherapist ever uses formal induction or the term *hypnosis*, imagery, relaxation, and suggestion can be invaluable adjunctive tools to one's practice.

Both hypnosis and hypnotic techniques are utilized within the context of the therapeutic relationship for symptom removal or modification, or for exploring issues when the process of therapy becomes blocked. Reduction of anxiety, development of self esteem, self awareness and ego strength and learning mechanisms for coping and conflict resolution are additional goals for these tools. Self regulation, biofeedback, adaptive escapism, and exploring creative and aesthetic avenues are potential results of hypnosis employed in a psychotherapeutic process (Singer and Pope, 1978). Hypnotic techniques promote the surfacing of unconscious materials so that both the client and therapist can gain insight and work toward change. "Imaginal techniques invite material that is likely to move selectively into the troubled areas of the client's life" (Klinger, 1980, p. 12). Imagery allows for articulation of problems and feelings when a patient is unable to express feelings verbally. Furthermore, if therapy becomes stalled because of resistance or verbal difficulties, hypnotic interventions can open up new paths of exploration in a manner that is often entertaining and nonthreatening. The symbols, patterns, and themes emerging from spontaneous imagery aid the therapist's and client's understanding of the problem. The techniques of dream enhancement, recall of important developmental incidents, and activation of transference speed and enrich the process of therapy.

The purposes of hypnosis and hypnotic techniques in psychotherapy and psychiatric nursing include the following:

- Reducing anxiety and stress
- Exploring possibilities when confronted with difficult decisions
- Altering psychosomatic symptoms
- Removing unwanted habits
- Building transference and a positive therapeutic relationship
- Regressing to past traumatic events for cartharsis and restructuring
- Eliminating blocks in the therapeutic process
- Controlling unwanted thoughts or perseverations
- Understanding unconscious processes

GROUP THERAPY TECHNIQUES AND HYPNOSIS

Much of the literature in hypnosis has focused on its use with individual patients. Recently, however, more attention has been paid to group and family work. Relaxation groups for stress management are common, as are short term groups for management of habit disorders. Smith (1982) studied college students in a workshop setting, using guided imagination in groups as an intervention for hopelessness. While the students reported improved study habits, the results were not statistically significant. The author noted that she measured short-term effects and the instruments might not have been sensitive.

In group and family psychotherapy these techniques can be utilized in several ways: as ice-breakers or warm-up exercises; to clarify issues as transference or questions of roles among group participants; to help individuals deal with a topic in a less restrictive and more creative manner.

THE PROCESS OF HYPNOSIS IN PSYCHOTHERAPY

The process of using hypnosis in the context of a therapeutic relationship is outlined in chapter one and applies to working with psychiatric patients as well. This process includes a clear definition of the problem, building a relationship of trust and positive expectation, devising a plan for intervention, intervening with the patient (in this case using some form of hypnosis), and evaluating the results in terms of the goals of therapy.

Because the word "hypnosis" carries mythology, adequate preparation of the patient is required when direct approaches are used (see chapter I and II). The advantage of labeling the intervention "hypnosis" is that the term often gives the patient the impression that something powerful is about to happen. Even when myths are discounted and disproved by the therapist, many continue believing in the magical potency of hypnosis. This, in itself, heightens the expectation that miraculous results can occur and may in and of itself create positive results. In some cases of negativism or severe resistence, however, unrealistic expectations can be detrimental: nothing is interpreted as successful and the patient loses faith in the intervention if anything less than total cure is experienced. Again this depends on the patient's personality dynamics, and the therapist needs to be sensitive to the individual's needs and styles of coping. To promote a positive outcome the therapist can indirectly suggest that results may be quick and dramatic, *or*, on the other hand, the process may take longer as the psyche evaluates the potential meaning of an outcome. The message given is that the wise unconscious will monitor the process. Permissive and vague suggestions about when a problem will be resolved, along with the emphasis that the problem *will* be resolved, benefits most types of patients. Interpreting results positively and correlating those results to the power within the patient decreases dependency on the therapist and fosters self-growth at the patient's own rate.

Imagery techniques, relaxation procedures, and direct and indirect suggestions without formal trance induction can all be used spontaneously without special preparation in a therapy session. The therapist can simply ask the patient to imagine a scene related to the problem presented, or to visualize the consequences of an action. Suggestions might be made subtly, such as, "Just as you solved a problem last week, so can you solve this current one," or more directly, "If you take your medication as prescribed you will begin to feel more in control."

The goals of psychotherapy vary with the individual and the problem presented. Overall, the therapeutic process, whether for increasing self-esteem, handling activities of daily living, or personality restructuring is activated and realized within the therapeutic relationship. This relationship is contractural whether or not a specific verbal agreement has been established: the patient comes, whether voluntarily or not, for help, and determining the best and most efficient means of intervention is the therapist's responsibility.

HYPNOTIC TECHNIQUES AND SYMPTOMS

According to Kroger and Fezler (1976), when people experience emotional problems they need to talk and want to be told what to do, particularly when they are anxious, confused, or depressed. They also need to be accepted as they are and to emancipate themselves from unduly dependent relationships (Kroger & Fezler, 1976). When dysfunction or illness develops, symptoms are symbolic representations of those unmet needs. Discord becomes a symptomatic defense against overwhelming feelings or actions. Nightmares, ideational problems, emotional discomfort, psychosomatic symptoms, and frank psychosis can all result.

Hypnotic techniques are often used to treat symptoms. Because symptoms have meaning and because the unconscious is "wise," difficulties sometimes stubbornly remain. A dynamic understanding and a tailored intervention are essential. Most often a permissive approach, utilizing the wisdom of the unconscious, is recommended when suggestions are given to explore or modify a problem. When the patient is in a relaxed (trance) state, the unconscious can be directed to work on an identified problem through dreams, either during sleep or trance. These dreams can inform the individual about the nature of the difficulty in tolerable doses of insight. Similarly, a therapist might instruct the individual's unconscious to survey his or her life and select the most relevant aspects for therapeutic work.

Many traditional therapists caution that the removal of a symptom with hypnosis is likely to disrupt the patient's defenses and exacerbate the illness. This may be true if the removal is premature. Symptom replacement and adverse reactions, when a symptom is eliminated in brief treatment with hypnosis, is not substantiated by research (Speigel, 1974). However, a needed symptom often becomes resistant to change. As generally believed in the practice of psychotherapy, if treatment occurs in a therapeutic relationship by a skilled, sensitive, and intelligent therapist, the patient is most likely to change at his or her own rate and without risk for further decompensation. The unconscious is "amazingly able to preserve the welfare of the self" (Stolzheise, 1961, p. 250).

THE DYNAMICS OF SYMPTOM DEVELOPMENT

How does the therapist accomplish a dynamic understanding of the problem? Many models for assessment exist. Cheek and LeCron (1968) and Edelstein (1981) outlined seven dynamics of symptom development that are helpful in hypnotic intervention.

Conflict. The basis of conflict is "I want—I can't or shouldn't have." The experience originates when we first do something to which our parents respond with "no." Conflicts producing symptoms frequently relate to sexual issues and to breaking (or to fear of breaking) moral codes. A symptom prevents action or wish fulfillment that is outside the individual's sense of right and wrong. A father loses his voice after yelling at his teenage daughter for leaving the house dressed in what he considers an overly seductive manner. He wants her to grow up, but at the same time does not want her seduced away from him by another man. Secretly he desires her for himself, but this desire is "unspeakable."

Motivation or Secondary Gain. Secondary gain is defined as the "external gain derived from any illness such as personal attention and service, monetary gains, disability benefits, and release from unpleasant responsibility" (*Psychiatric Glossary*, 1980, p. 122). Primary gain, on the other hand, is obtaining "relief from emotional *conflict* and the freedom from *anxiety* achieved by a *defense mechanism*" (*Psychiatric Glossary*, 1980, p. 109). Both are closely related to unconscious processes and are seldom understood consciously by the individual. Does the symptom serve a special purpose? Many symptoms, no matter how unpleasant, provide reward. Chronic pain, for example, allows one to remain on workmen's compensation (a secondary gain). Sometimes the reward is not concrete, but only promised. For example, a woman so anxious about upcoming surgery as to be nearly phobic, was hoping that if she died, her mother would feel sad and regret previous mistreatment (again, secondary gain).

Identification. The client identifies strongly with a person and develops the same problem that the identified-with person has. Even a hated parent can become the object of identification. For example, a daughter who becomes obese like her mother, and the son who becomes alcoholic like his father, both despised their parent's "failings" but identified unconsciously and incorporated the same problems.

Masochism. The aims of self-punishment are to avoid punishment from others and to relieve guilt. LeCron and Cheek (1968) explained that sometimes one part of the unconscious will compliment an unacceptable behavior while the other part demands punishment for the transgression. Insight is seldom sufficient to solve the problem. Behavior change is needed in addition to finding new ways to meet old needs.

Imprint. An imprint is "an idea that has become fixed in the subconscious part of the mind and then is carried out in the exact same way as a posthypnotic suggestion" (Cheek & LeCron, 1968, p. 98). Many maladaptive symptoms are compulsive acting-out of an old message that was long ago forgotten. A health care professional telling a newly diagnosed cancer patient, "You will never get over this" can lead to the patient totally giving up. A patient who feels no options exist and holds firmly to that symptom was probably told there was no way out at a previous stressful time.

Organ or Body Language. The psychological symptom is transformed into a physical problem. A psychophysiological (psychosomatic) symptom is a symbolic representation of feelings the individual can't express directly (Edelstein, 1981). (A young man had chronic diarrhea which was progressing to colitis. As we talked he mentioned that he and his lover had broken up. He couldn't "stomach" how he had been treated any longer, but now he was lonely and having second thoughts about breaking up the relationship.)

Past Experience. The symptom or problem in this category results from an actual experience, rather than from something the client was told. He or she anticipates that similar experiences will produce the same results. New situations are reacted to with the same behavior and feelings, although these new situations may not, on surface examination, resemble the initial experience. (See "Phobia" later in this chapter.)

These dynamics are useful in conceptualizing patient's problems and may also be employed in the intervention through ideomotor signaling (finger signals to answer questions) as an uncovering technique in psychotherapy.

SELECTION OF APPROPRIATE PATIENTS FOR HYPNOSIS

Because of the dissociation and the potential emergence of unconscious material, hypnotic techniques are not usually recommended with patients who are psychotic, severely borderline, in marginal control, depressed, or suicidal. Using hypnosis with depressed patients has been controversial. Crasilneck and Hall (1975) explained that the dynamics of suicidal ideation relate most often to intense anger. When the depression is of a reactive nature, the anger is usually directed toward a recent disappointment. In cases of more severe depression, however, the anger is usually connected with repressed infantile rage. Hypnosis moves a patient rapidly into situations involving transference distortions, and if a depressed suicidal patient experiences a real or imagined slight from the therapist, the punishment for the therapist might be the patient's suicide. Other authors, however, contend that hypnotic techniques are successful and safe with depressed patients. Singer and Pope (1978) contend that imagery with mildly depressed individuals breaks up the "snowball effect" of depression by allowing for a relaxed, pleasurable experience. Schultz (1978) found short-term positive effects of imagery with a male, severely depressed, hospitalized population. These patients imagined pleasant positive scenes, improved self-images, and were then more capable of positive emotions and laughter.

The techniques described throughout this book aim to help the patient feel more in control and to build ego strength. Indirect suggestion and the use of imagery without formal trance induction can be useful with most, including psychotic and suicidal patients. Suicidal patients, for example, are often asked during assessment to picture and describe what they think will happen after they die. Such information can aid understanding of the dynamics of the suicidal ideation and subsequently enhance the evaluation of potential lethality. Similarly these techniques can be used for ego building with psychotic and borderline patients.

Clients who are organically impaired (retarded, senile, demented, etc.) rarely can concentrate for sufficient amounts of time and often have such trouble with memory and cognition that these techniques are not always useful. Brief relaxation exercises, positive suggestions, and simple images certainly can be employed and often yield positive results. Reminiscing with the elderly is a good example of an effective use of imagery with a potentially organically impaired population. Techniques have also been developed to work with the blind and deaf and appear on occasion in the literature.

HYPNOSIS FOR ANXIETY AND STRESS REDUCTION*

A college student volunteered to be a subject for demonstration during a class on hypnotic techniques. She explained she was unable to relax and as a result had numerous psychosomatic problems, including a spastic colon and a developing peptic ulcer. In addition to her college studies she had a demanding job and a family. Her stress was becoming so intense that she was unable to concentrate. She became disoriented, sometimes getting off the subway several stops before or after her own. She couldn't keep her hands still; her thoughts raced. She wanted relief but was afraid to relax because she might go to sleep and lose hours of valuable work time. I asked her how she had in the past been able to relax. She had enjoyed physical exercise but now could not find the time. I asked if she had any questions or concerns about hypnosis. She did not and was enthusiastic about trying it. I told her to sit comfortably and close her eyes. I asked if for "just a bit" she could focus her attention on her hands.

I described various sensations, such as warmth, tingling, and numbness, that she "might" be feeling. The feeling "might" be like having on "big space gloves." I encouraged her to experience the sensations and to realize that she was having the pleasant sensations because she was relaxed and had focused her attention. I told her she was doing well and looked more relaxed. I then asked her to focus on only one finger—I gave here the posthypnotic suggestion that she would be able to focus on that finger or her hands whenever and wherever she wanted, and that when she did this she would experience relaxation and relief in a short period of time. After reorienting to usual awareness, the client stated she felt good and more relaxed. I encouraged her to do this brief exercise a couple of times a day, and she agreed since it was *brief*.

I chose this highly focused method because this client reported that her thoughts raced and her concentration was poor. Using a defined, circumscribed, and sensitive part of her body (her hands and one finger) helped her control her thinking and had potential for success. She told me she liked physical exercise, so a *physical* sensation was utilized rather than an imaginary scene. Because this woman was obsessive, clearly overextended, and fearful of not meeting numerous demands, she needed to experience relief through a brief, succinct process. A lengthy progressive relaxation exercise might have made her more anxious and decreased the likelihood that she would practice. I

---

*All the case examples used in this chapter are drawn from psychiatric nursing practice.

emphasized, as a result she would, because of a simple relaxation technique, have more control over her life.

TRANSFERENCE AND RELATIONSHIP BUILDING
WITH A DEPRESSED PATIENT

Nel experienced periods of depression and hopelessness about her future. During our first several sessions, she sat nearly nonverbal, with her arms angrily folded. She described feeling isolated and hopeless about her future because of physical problems. I had to ask several questions to elicit the simplest response. I commented that she looked angry, which she denied. Feeling at an impasse, one day I asked her to close her eyes, relax, and picture what was going on. I did no formal induction of hypnosis and indeed never used the word because I felt she would have been frightened and even more resistant. Nel did not look particularly relaxed using the imagery, which took about five minutes. When I asked her to tell me what she was experiencing, she described being on an island alone. Weighted down by heavy chains, she was becoming increasingly tired. The tide was coming in and she knew she could not float or swim to shore. I asked if she could see people on the shore who might come help her; she stated there were but they couldn't make it in time. I asked her if she could see a boat that might rescue her. There was one, but it was too far away to reach her. The water was getting deeper; she knew she was going to drown. I suggested she see me on the shore and that I could come help her. She said, "No, you're not a good swimmer." I asked her to open her eyes. Clearly she was experiencing the scene vividly and was tense and anxious. She stated she really was hopeless and helpless. I commented that it didn't seem she felt I could help her either, and she agreed. I explained that I did think help was available, but she would have to avail herself of it by visualizing that help.

The next session she arrived looking much brighter. She opened the session saying, "You know, the strangest thing happened to me on the bus on the way home last week. I kept having this image pop into my head of my drowning in the water, but you were swimming out to get me. You had flippers and goggles on and you were a *very good* swimmer. You got to me and rescued me." I questioned what she thought that all meant. She replied, "I don't know but I felt better." I asked her if it might mean that she felt more hopeful and that I could help her even when things seemed desperate. She agreed this might be possible.

Nel had been extremely isolated when therapy began. She had felt betrayed by all her friends when she needed them the most. A frequent theme when she experienced similar depressions was that she was alone, maligned, mistreated, and there was no hope for her situation to ever change. She was angry but feared her anger. Even though she was often provocative, she dreaded others' anger, anticipating ultimate rejection. Often she entertained thoughts of being better off dead than alive. In such condition, she communicated little verbally. This behavior probably replicated times when she was a very small, nearly nonverbal child and experienced her mother's rejection when she was ill and very much in need of her attention. Often Nel's symptoms were minimized by her mother, and expressing her feelings was discouraged.

The imagery technique provided a nonverbal opportunity for Nel to picture how she felt, allowing her to intensify the feeling and gain new understanding. Her resistance to trusting me and her fear of closeness were clearly heard in her statement, "You're not a very good swimmer." Consciously she was angry, but unconsciously she wanted to trust me and believe I had the power to rescue her. This was demonstrated by the image which spontaneously appeared later. This brief exercise broke through three weeks of depression and hopelessness and was attempted after rational and logical means were unsuccessful.

CONFLICT, RESOLUTION, AND DECISION-MAKING

Psychotherapy clients frequently present with conflicts over major and minor life decisions. Many techniques are available for helping individuals resolve such issues. Relaxation followed by imagining alternatives, and ego-building suggestions that the individual has the power to make the right decisions, are frequently employed, with or without hypnosis.

Pat, a 36-year-old man, had worked for many years in an institution where he felt abused and unappreciated. Although dissatisfied with his job and profession, he felt unable, at this point in his life, to make a major career change. Whatever he wanted to do, he knew he needed to return to school, but, single and self-supporting, Pat felt unable to attend school full-time and that it would take the rest of his life to get a degree. He stated that he was "on the fence." The issue of job and career change had been a consistent theme throughout therapy. The unresolved conflict clearly related to many issues, including success versus failure and independence versus dependence.

Without a formal induction, I asked Pat to close his eyes and imagine his situation. He clearly saw himself sitting not on a fence, but on a rough log so large that he could not straddle it comfortably. A safe height off the ground, he did not feel in danger. He could clearly see the vista in front of him: green bush grass that was scraggly rather than lush. To find out what was behind him would have been uncomfortable and might cause him to fall off the log. When encouraged to speculate what might be in back of him, Pat had no fantasy. He opened his eyes and explained that his present situation (sitting on the fence), while unpleasant was easier than facing the unknown. This metaphor aptly described how frightening it was for Pat to change.

After this intervention, some behavior changes began to occur. Pat informed his supervisor that if he was sent to one particular place again he would leave his job; he also attended a workshop specifically related to members of his profession who wanted to change careers. A few months later he re-enrolled in school.

Dolly, a 28-year-old single woman, related discomfort in her inability to finish her doctoral dissertation. If she didn't complete this paper she would forfeit her degree for another year. While describing the situation, she smiled and looked coquettish, almost as if she was daring me to confront her or tell her directly what to do. Many aspects of the conflict existed. She wanted the degree but was disillusioned with her profession and not sure that she wanted to continue. If she wanted to achieve her goal of teaching, she need the Ph.D. degree, but what she wanted most was to marry and have children. Her fiancé was highly accomplished, intellectual, and could not understand why she didn't finish; she felt inferior to him and to his astounding ability to accumulate degrees in various fields. Furthermore, she insisted the demands of her advisor regarding the paper were unreasonable. She stated in a whining voice, "I just don't want to do it." Both parents had died within the last six years. When asked what they would advise her, she quickly stated they would undoubtedly tell her to finish no matter what else she wanted to do. I asked her to do an exercise to help clarify the conflict and then help her find the solution. I chose the inner dialogue technique without formal hypnotic induction.

When I asked Dolly to close her eyes she initially resisted, but then giggled and complied. Then I said, "You have a conflict, and the two sides can have a conversation in your head. Listen to what both sides say. What does the side that wants you to finish the paper say and how does it sound? (pause) Does it sound like anyone you know? (pause) Now listen to the side that doesn't want you to finish. (pause) What does that side sound like? What does it say?" (pause) She was restless and said, "Do I have to keep my eyes closed?" I told her she could do what she liked and what was right for her. I continued. "You know you have a third part that is your creative part, and I bet that part can come up with a more innovative solution for you. That part can work for you both on a conscious and unconscious level and will let you know what to do soon." She opened her eyes and was slightly tearful. She explained she had always been very bright; school work had been easy. She never had to work until this graduate program to get good grades. She felt her potential and creativity had been wasted; she was now too old to change her path and all was lost. She explained that the voices in her head were hard to hear, but the part that wanted to finish sounded like her parents and the part that didn't, a young version of herself. Her parents had always encouraged her and expected her to do well in school. At the same time, she was told that women did not have careers and should be at home, married and raising children. When she decided on a profession, they did not support either a career or her choice of profession. While at this point the conflict was not solved, an emotional reaction had occurred, which clarified some of the issues.

Dolly came to her next appointment looking more relaxed but still somewhat coquettish and furtive. She had decided to write her paper and had talked with her instructor. She was going to finish. I asked how she decided this; she answered she didn't know. She had done some reading over the weekend and felt she could finish the paper soon, although no deadline had been set. She had followed all of my indirect suggestions. She was still, however, not sure what she wanted to do with her life or what kind of work she might like to pursue. I mentioned again that she had reacted to the exercise by feeling that her creative and intellectual abilities had not been realized. The remainder of the session focused on parental expectations and her desires for a "good life." Strong dependency needs and anger at her parents became clear, as well as feelings of unrealized potential.

THE ACTING-OUT OR DISRUPTIVE PATIENT

When a crisis is brewing and a patient's behavior begins to escalate, our adrenaline and sympathetic nervous system become activated. Unconsciously we model the patient and develop a stress reaction ourselves. Nurses, particularly on inpatient psychiatric units, deal with patients who become overwhelmed with feelings and lose control over their behavior. Clearly these incidents are dangerous for both patient and staff, and limits must be imposed. Both verbal methods and body language can promote a successful outcome. The nurse must first establish self-control. Taking a moment for a deep breath, dropping the shoulders to relieve tension, and saying to oneself, "I can handle this situation in a positive manner" takes only a moment and can make the difference between the patient's becoming dangerous or going into an environment of reduced stimulation relatively cooperatively. Saying, as you escort the patient to the "quiet room" or are giving a medication, "As you relax you will be less upset; I am a nurse and am going to help you feel better. As I give you medication you will feel more relaxed, and as you relax and rest you will gain more control and feel better. You will feel more secure and your thoughts will slow down. Things will become more clear to you as you relax. You can help this process by cooperating and trying to breathe more easily and regularly. Breathe slowly and regularly as I inject this medication. The medication will help you regain control." (Note the use of "as" rather than "if." "As" communicates the expectation of a positive outcome.) These words can be modified depending on the patient and the situation. If your voice is kept slow and easy, the instructions are repeated, and you connect relaxation and cooperation with increased comfort and control, the patient is more likely to regain control quickly.

HYPNOTIC TECHNIQUES TO CLARIFY THE PROCESS OF THERAPY

During therapy it is not uncommon for the therapist and patient to wonder where they are in the overall process. Sometimes patients begin to appear stuck and present less material during sessions. While this may be a therapeutic impasse, it may also indicate that the patient is getting better and termination is approaching. Both therapist and patient may avoid this, not wanting to separate or not trusting that in fact most of the issues that brought the person into treatment have been resolved. Dreams, fantasies and preoccupations with or without the hypnotic state can also clarify where the therapist and patient are in the process.

Betty had been in therapy over a year. She came specifically for hypnosis because she was unable to make decisions in her life. Twenty-five years old, she was still living with her parents, was unable to leave a job she hated or her boyfriend, to whom she no longer felt attracted and who also lived with her and her parents. She was dependent and felt stuck in her negative feelings. We used hypnosis to uncover her motivations for such strong dependency needs, as well as ego-building techniques so she could feel strong enough to make rational decisions.

Finally she planned to leave her job and informed her boyfriend that he had to either get a job or leave her parents' house. Soon after these decisions, she reported in a session that when she practiced self-hypnosis she saw my face and heard my voice. I interpreted this as transference of dependency from her parents to me. She also described a recent dream. She was in a large cave and was about to experience an important event, or ritual. She was wrapped in a shroud and was about to be submerged in water attended by several old crones and me. They told her, "you have done your job and now you can have your bath." She was placed on a movable slab and slid into the water. She was submerged but felt secure and comfortable. During the therapy session she redreamed the dream in hypnosis, and I suggested that her unconscious could help her understand the meaning more fully. Afterward I asked if she had been feeling depressed, thinking that the shroud and the ritual might indicate death or a death wish. She denied this and insisted that she had accomplished something and was being rewarded rather than punished. She felt hopeful and excited rather than depressed. It became increasingly clear that the dream related more to rebirth than to death. When I asked her about this she stated it was indeed true that she was feeling like a new person, stronger and more capable of making important changes in her life. This clarified more than a lengthy discussion where she was in the process of therapy. She terminated in the next few weeks and as far as I know is still doing well.

PHOBIA

Phobia, as defined by the DSM III (1980), is a "persistent irrational fear of a specific object, activity or situation that results in a compelling desire to avoid" the phobic stimulus. The individual recognizes the fear as irrational and out of proportion to the actual danger, and normal behavior is impeded as a result of the fear. Interestingly, the individual experiencing extreme stress often enters a "trance-like state" as a coping mechanism for the panic (Frankel, 1974).

Hypnosis has often been utilized either as a primary form of treatment or as an adjunctive process to other forms of treatment. Wolpe (1966) described systematic desensitization and flooding for phobias; both techniques utilized relaxation training, imagery, and often hypnosis. "Restructuring" for phobias was outlined by Spiegel (1978). In this technique neither the reasons for nor the consequences of the phobia are emphasized. Rather, the individual's limitations and strengths are noted and reformulated with the emphasis on potential ways of "integrating motivation with consequences." An old problem is subsequently approached in a new framework. The trance encourages intense focal awareness which implies that the individual can synthesize and integrate thought, feeling, and behavior.

Behavioral rehearsal, ego-building suggestions, and inner advisor techniques are also often incorporated into the process. Often working to end a phobia takes place within the context of longer-term, dynamically oriented psychotherapy. Hypnotic age regression to relive the original trauma can be one approach. Achieving a relatively deep hypnotic state is necessary when age regression, automatic writing, or hypnotic dream work is used (Mott, 1981).

Case Example: Phobia

Mary, a young mother of two children, was phobic of thunderstorms. She was uncomfortable in enclosed spaces, particularly when riding in a car on the highway with the windows up. She was extremely fearful of being alone at night, and since her husband traveled this caused her difficulty.

She had been in psychotherapy and was very bright, verbal, insightful, and motivated to both understand and resolve the phobia. She knew about hypnosis, had no fear of it, and came to therapy requesting that be the modality. She had also used the Lamaze method (a technique similar to hypnosis; see chapter 9) successfully for the birth of her two children.

During the history-taking, the potential causes for and a complete description of the symptom was obtained. She related that her mother had always been fearful of thunderstorms and described an incident when she was 10 of being in an auditorium with a cousin during a severe thunderstorm; both she and her cousin had been frightened. When her grandfather had died several years ago, she could not be reached right away; she thought this incident also might be associated with her phobia as his death happened on a weekend when the news reported thunderstorms and a tornado unexpectedly striking a New England town. Her fears had intensified when as an adult she and her family began spending time at a seaside summer cottage where thunderstorms were common.

Mary described her symptom as follows; I can see the thunderstorms building on the horizon and worry they might become tornados. I feel vulnerable and out of control. When I hear on the radio thunderstorms are predicted my anxiety begins to build. I watch as the clouds increase and darken. If I notice thunderheads at the beach I quickly pack up the children and go home. I put the porch furniture away and, once in the house, close all the windows. All these preparations heighten my sense of impending doom. When the thunderstorm hits, I panic, feeling my stomach knotting.

Because of childhood illness one leg had been amputated below the knee when Mary was 11 years old. While she felt she adjusted to that loss through prior psychotherapy, I suspected this was a highly traumatic event and might be related to her present phobia.

First Session

We agreed to use hypnosis and a desensitization model. In a relaxed state, Mary could comfortably encounter thunderstorms through imagery. When she became anxious, she was to let me know by raising a finger on her *left* hand; I would help her relax again before we proceeded; she could let me know she was comfortable by raising a finger on her *right* hand. She chose to lay down on a couch and quickly entered trance while listening to gentle rhythmic speech and suggestions of deep relaxation. I told her we could recreate her experience with thunderstorms while she was in this nice comfortable state. I encouraged her unconscious mind to help her understand the symptom if, and when, it would be helpful to her. I told her she was a good hypnotic subject; she had experienced deep relaxation in the past with Lamaze, and she could do that again *now*. I then said, "See yourself on the beach near your cottage. You heard in the morning that thunderstorms were predicted, and as you look off in the distance you see the clouds building; you hear the distant rumble of thunder, and you see small flashes of lightning. (Her breathing had quickened, but she did not raise a finger to inform me of discomfort, so I continued.) Because a thunderstorm appears likely, you begin to pack up all the beach stuff and to gather the kids together." (She raised a finger and appeared even more uncomfortable.) I encouraged her to take a deep breath and to relax her stomach muscles and to re-experience her nice sense of relaxation. Since there was little remaining time in the session, I helped her dehypnotize by counting to five and suggesting she would be comfortable and relaxed and we could continue to work on this problem. I offered her posthypnotic suggestions for comfort and said her unconscious mind would continue to be her friend and helper. She would learn what she needed to know.

Mary explained after the hypnosis that she was anxious when she saw the clouds building but became *very* anxious when packing up. She looked surprised for a moment and stated, "You know, it reminded me of packing to go to the Mayo Clinic for tests when I was 3 or 4. I was also very anxious about the darkening sky. It looked like a band of darkness closing in on me. It sounds maybe trite, but it seemed like having an anesthesia mask put over me. Do you think that's possible?" I replied it was possible and that her illness and surgery must have been very frightening. We talked about how hard it was for her then to understand all that was happening, and told her that we would talk more about it the next session.

Second Session

Mary felt confused about how the thunderstorm phobia could be related to her hospitalizations. Tearful, she expressed concern about losing her defenses. I told her again that she was in charge and need only go as fast as was tolerable, learning only what she needed. During the trance that day, I used ego-strengthening suggestions of ability to grow, develop, and gain control of her feelings. I emphasized relaxation and comfort. While she again experienced anxiety visualizing the sky darkening, she was able to relax when encouraged to do so.

Third Session

Mary wanted to get to the bottom of all this, but she was not sure why she felt the amputation and surgery were related to the phobia. Generally she felt better; she had comfortably ridden in a car on the highway, and for the first time she was more at ease when she was home alone. During trance, I suggested that she experience any incidents related to the thunderstorm anxiety and that the meaning of symbols would become more clear to her. The guided imagery in the trance was, "You are at the cottage. It's morning and you hear on the radio thunderstorms are predicted. As the day progresses, you look out the back door and see the sky darken and the clouds build. The wind is blowing harder and the air is changing in temperature. You can smell the distant rain.

Thunder is getting louder and the lighning closer. You are closing the windows." She raised her finger, indicating discomfort. I suggested she could talk if she wanted about what was happening. She appeared to be having some trouble breathing and was crying. She described the darkness as oppressive; she felt very alone and frightened. She said, "I've been such a good girl; how can you do this to me?" When she seemed to have finished crying, I encouraged her to deeply relax again and then helped her dehypnotize with suggestions that she was doing well and learning about herself and her problem.

Sad and frightened during the trance, Mary told me that she experienced the darkness and the approaching thunderstorm with relative comfort but with a feeling of being "closed in"; also the "windows" bothered her. She sensed her feelings were related to the surgery. Her amputation had been discussed very little and she had never cried about it. Now she talked at length about the experience, how badly her mother and father felt and how intent she was on walking soon on the prosthesis. She described herself as a very good child. Now she was aware that at the time she felt unjustifiably punished. Now she was feeling some relief, although she continued to be having some difficulty breathing. I encouraged her to take some nice deep breaths and to close her eyes if she wished, which she did. I suggested relaxation and comfort and, again, that what she was learning would be very helpful to her.

Fourth Session

During the next week Mary felt better. She thought her problem breathing was like being intubated in the recovery room; difficulty breathing was a common feeling when she was phobic and was also related to trying not to cry. During the trance, she managed to have comfort throughout the thunderstorm. She was aware of tension when the windows were mentioned and described what she saw in her imagination: "There are lights around the windows like circles. I want to go back and experience what happened the night before the surgery." (I encouraged her to do that.) "I'm very alone and scared. I can't sleep. My mother isn't here and I want her. The woman in the next bed is talking to me; she's sitting with me and holding my hand. I finally go to sleep. I don't know how." I said, "Do you want to go to the next day?"

"Yes. They've given me medicine, and I'm sleepy; my mouth is so dry. They take me to the operating room and I have to wait a long time outside. I'm there so long. I keep falling asleep. I'm strapped down, and I want to run. They take me in finally and strap me to the table. I want to run so bad, but I'm strapped down, and I'm so sleepy and groggy. There's a big round circle of light above my head." (She is tearful and sobbing.) I asked her what she was feeling. "Scared. I want my mother! . . . The anesthesiologist lets me take the anesthesia gently holding the side of my head. I went to sleep."

At this point, she appeared calm. I encouraged her to relax even more and to be comfortable. I stated that remembering all this pain would help her in many aspects of her life; her unconscious was letting her know a great deal and could continue to do so in doses that were tolerable to her. After the trance, she stated she felt cleansed and good, and she felt no more need to cry.

Fifth Session

Mary reported three dreams she thought might be related. These are brief descriptions of those dreams.

DREAM 1.   I'm in a big room with two blond curly-headed boys that are not my own. There is another helping woman present. There is a concrete floor and two big tubs. They need a bath and the tubs are being filled with water. We can't stop the water; the tubs are overflowing and we're afraid we'll drown. Suddenly I see a door and open it. It's a bathroom, kind of like the one here. It has a drain in the floor, and I pull the plug. All the water drains out and we're saved."

Therapist's Interpretation: The two boys might have resembled two parts of her personality: one who wants to be cleansed of her feelings, and the other who is fearful of the flood of emotion and tears. That part is afraid of drowning. A female caretaker was present, which might have been me. Mary herself found the drain, which saved them all from drowning. Even with the flood of emotion, she was strong enough to save all of them.

DREAM 2.   "Another blond curly-haired boy, who this time resembles a child I know, has climbed up into a storage area I have. I asked him to come down, but he wouldn't. He was gleeful and devilish. He was throwing all kinds of things down— suitcases of old clothes and things I hadn't been able to find including a garbage bag full of things. He was resistant but having such a good time."

Therapist's Interpretation: Mary had described that while the process of treatment was painful it was exciting and even intellectually stimulating. She had some need to resist but at the same time a need to get rid of "old stuff." When she mentioned the garbage bag, my fantasy was of how the amputated leg—a valuable part of her—had probably been discarded in a garbage bag. When I asked her about the garbage bag, she had no associations.

DREAM 3.   "I'm in an amphitheater that's surrounded by hills. My mother is on the top of the hill. I'm trying to climb the hill to get to her, but I can't get to her. I feel if I can't get to her, she will be lost forever. This [dream] was sad and upsetting."

Therapist's Interpretation: The amphitheater clearly replicated the operating amphitheater. Her mother was not allowed to be with her; Mary felt deserted and that she would never see her again. In addition, she could not climb the hill easily with her withered leg, but she felt no hope existed once the leg was amputated.

We discussed the three dreams. I emphasized the hopeful quality of the first two, that although Mary was reliving a frightening experience she was doing well. One thunderstorm had occurred recently, to which she reacted with only minor anxiety. She continued to be more comfortable alone and driving in an enclosed car.

Several aspects of the phobia had become clear to both of us. The loss of control and sense of vulnerability experienced during a storm was probably related to Mary's inability to prevent the loss of her leg. A thunderstorm is violent, unpredictable, and can cause harm and even kill. She had the same dread about the amputation but had not resolved it. Even though simple desensitization in a trance state had been attempted, she had age-regressed spontaneously and related the phobia and the amputation. She wanted to explore this further. What seemed missing was grief resolution for her leg and anger at both the people involved and at having had to experience such trauma.

When I asked Mary how she felt about the amputated leg, she replied it had to come off; it was withered; as she grew it did not. She couldn't wear a shoe as the toes were twisted and curled under, and her walking ability had become seriously compromised. I asked what she thought had been done with the leg. She stated it was probably just disposed of. When queried further if that was what she would have wanted, she was quiet for a moment and then she stated, "No. I wish it had been buried."

During the usual trance induction utilizing the same imagery, she began talking about the blackness of the storm. "As I look at the blackness and the clouds, I can see clearly it's a tornado coming. My God, the funnel of the tornado is black and the shape of a boot. It's my withered leg!" I asked her to see it very clearly, than gradually to see the "tornado" leg change. "If you are ready to let it go, let the blackness become lighter in color until it turns grey. Let it move off into the distance slowly and peacefully, its color changing and the grey melding into pink; it's fading calmly and peacefully, and it can disappear or become a tiny speck off in the distance if you like." I hoped this would provide symbolic burial.

Following dehypnotization, she described the experience as "incredible." She was elated with a touch of sadness. "The tornado is my leg. I turned rosy pink and got very calm and small. It did disappear. I feel much better; I'm drained."

Sixth Session

Mary looked like a storm cloud. She had been cranky and ill-tempered all week. She had to get to the anger of the storm; the storm was within her. She described the doctor who performed the amputation as a kindly old gentleman who clearly did not want to hurt her and was not happy about amputating her leg. I mentioned it must have been hard to be angry with him, particularly since he was so kind. She was also angry with her mother for not being there even though she was not allowed, and for not encouraging her to express her feelings. During the trance I encouraged her to say, either aloud or silently, whatever she wanted to those at whom she was angry. She called the doctor a "bastard"; she said she wanted to claw their eyes out, bite and stab them with knives. She felt the storm subside and looked calm, but then the storm built again. Her breathing increased and she looked agitated and uncomfortable. She heard the saw in the distance, about to amputate her leg. She cried, "How can you do this awful thing to me! I've been such a good girl. I don't deserve this. I want to kill you. I hear all those voices yelling, but not at me." She calmed again, and I encouraged her to continue being calm and relaxed, to let today's storm subside. She was able to get relaxed and comfortable with no obvious signs of the "storm" brewing again. I encouraged this because the session was almost over and because it seemed to be enough catharsis. She stated that hearing the saw was awful but that venting the anger was helpful.

Seventh Session

Mary recalled a dream she had as a child shortly after she came home from the surgery. She was being attacked by Indians with arrows and knives. The lightning, she said, is the arrows and knives; the thunder is all those voices yelling. The voices are probably symbolic of her own need to express anger, and the knives are clearly the symbol of her torture and mutilation and desire to retaliate. She had continued to be cranky all week; there was more anger to get out. We had only two more sessions, since she was leaving for her cottage for the summer. She felt the pressure of time and was very motivated to finish. During the trance, I again encouraged her to re-experience whatever she needed to rid herself of the anger. Again she saw the doctor and again she attacked him. When the storm subsided, I asked if she could put all of her feelings into a symbol or an object. She could see a big, ugly, brown-and-black blob. She stabbed and kicked "it." She saw herself on a bridge with "it." I asked her what she wanted to do with it. She said, "It's too heavy to lift, but I think I can push it off the side. It's sliding off the edge. It's floating out to sea." I asked if it still looked the same. "No. It changed mass and shape. It's floating on the top. It sparkles like egg white. It's just floating farther and farther away." I then encouraged her to go to her cottage and to sit in it feeling calm and peaceful. She was now safe and secure. Didn't she think so? She answered, "Yes."

Mary spent a much more comfortable summer at her cottage, even though it was a summer of frequent, exceptionally violent, dangerous thunderstorms.

As is often the case with psychotherapy, an interesting spinoff occurred. Mary shared detailed information about her experience in hypnosis with her husband. She later related that they wept as she described her pain, isolation, and fear. He understood her rage and her previous anxiety when he was away. She felt they were much closer as a result.

Discussion

Working with Mary was an emotionally exciting and gratifying experience. Her courage and ability to deal with the stress of the actual amputation, as well as her willingness to experience it again through hypnosis must be acknowledged. Seldom do therapists have such motivated and insightful patients. It must also be noted that I knew Mary prior to the initiation of treatment, and we had discussed in brief the difficulties a child encounters when hospitalized. As mentioned, she was well-schooled in its theories. As a result, effort and time that normally would have been necessary to establish trust and alleviate fears and misconceptions were not needed except as issues came up during the process.

Mary spontaneously regressed in hypnosis to the hospital experience. This may happen with other patients, and the therapist must be prepared. It need not be a frightening experience for either therapist or patient if it is framed in a positive way; the patient is reminded that the experience can promote growth and that the subconscious should only confront painful issues in amounts that are tolerable. When such intense reactions occur, patients often experience amnesia or selective recall. This is protective and the patient can be encouraged over time to gradually integrate the content in whatever way is appropriate. Mary also started dreaming and wrote those dreams down so they could be discussed during the next session. Re-dreaming in hypnosis could have been useful but did not seem necessary, since in the nontrance normal state she was able to discuss their meaning and apply it to the problem. If therapy had been blocked or resistance had become a problem, the use of these dreams through re-dreaming them in hypnosis could have helped move the treatment along.

SUMMARY

These case examples describe many potential uses of hypnosis in psychiatric nursing practice. Some examples involved specific inductions of a hypnotic state, while others were incorporated without any formal induction into the normal process of therapy. Because these techniques may speed up the process and allow insight, the clinician is cautioned to utilize ego-building and supportive techniques whenever uncovering techniques are considered. The availability of a competent consultant is often useful. As adverse reactions are uncommon, the skilled clinician should consider using these techniques to aid the process of therapy. Surprising changes in behavior and affect may be the result, even when a patient is unable to verbally describe psychological insight. Indeed, the examples in all the chapters of the book describe the use of hypnotic techniques as part of a therapeutic process oriented toward promoting growth, comfort, and increased self-esteem.

REFERENCES

Cheek, D.B., & LeCron, L.M. (1968). *Clinical hypnotherapy*. New York: Grune & Stratton.

Crasilneck, H.B., & Hall, J.A. (1975). *Clinical hypnosis: Principles and applications*. New York: Grune & Stratton.

Diagnostic and Statistical Manual of Mental Disorders (DSMII) (3rd Ed.) (1981). American Psychiatric Association. Washington, D.C.

Edelstein, M.J. (1981). *Trauma, trance and transformation: A clinical guide to psychotherapy*. New York: Brunner/Mazel.

Frankel, F.H. (1956). Trance capacity and the genesis of phobic reactions. In LeCron, L.M. (Ed.), *Experimental hypnosis*. New York: Macmillan.

Klinger, E. (1980). Therapy and the flow of thought. In Shorr, J.E., Sobel, G.E., Robin, P., & Connelly, J.A. (Eds.). *Imagery: Its many dimensions and implications*. New York: Plenum.

Kroger, W.S., & Fezler, W.D. (1976). *Hypnosis and behavior modification: Imagery conditioning*. Philadelphia: J.B. Lippincott.

Mott, T. (1981). Hypnosis and phobic disorders. *Psychiatric Annals, 11*, 36–45.

Peplau, H. (1982). Therapeutic concepts. In Smoyak, S. and Rouslin, S. (Eds.) *A collection of classics in psychiatric nursing literature*. New Jersey: Charles B. Slack (originally published 1957).

American Psychiatric Association. (1980). *A psychiatric glossary* (5th Ed.) (1980). Boston: Little Brown.

Rogers, M.E. (1970). *An introduction to the theoretical basis of nursing*. Philadelphia: F.A. Davis.

Shultz, D. (1978). Imagery and the control of depression. In Singer, J.L., & Pope, K.S. (Eds.). *The power of human imagination*. New York: Plenum.

Singer, J.L., & Pope, K.S. (1978). *The power of human imagination*. New York: Plenum.

Singer, J.L. (1974). *Imagery and daydream methods in psychotherapy and behavior modification*. New York: Academic Press.

Smith, D.M.Y. (1982). Guided imagination as an intervention in hopelessness. *Journal of Psychiatric Nursing and Mental Health Services, 20*, 29–32.

Spiegel, H., & Rockey, E. (1974). Hypnosis in surgery: exploding the myths. *The Surgical Team, 3*, 31–37 (Reprinted in Nursing Digest, March-April, 1975).

Spiegel, H., & Spiegel, D. (1978). *Trance and treatment*. New York: Basic Books.

Stolzhiese, R.M. (1961). Psychotherapy simplified. In LeCron, L. (Ed.). *Techniques of hypnotherapy*. New York: Julian Press.

Wolpe, J., & Lazarus, A.A. (1966). *Behavior therapy techniques: A guide to the treatment of neuroses*. New York: Pergamon Press.

Zahourek, R.P. (1982). Hypnosis in nursing practice: Emphasis on the patient who has pain—part I and II. *Journal of Psychiatric Nursing and Mental Health Services, 20*, 13–17; 21–24.

Appendix

The following are examples of inductions. Each clinician will find an individual style, a favorite induction and become sensitive to the kind of induction that is most likely to be successful with a given individual. These are largely direct suggestive and induction techniques. Indirect techniques are exemplified in chapters 2, 3 and 13. Additional examples of indirect suggestive techniques and an Ericksonian induction appear later in this appendix.

PROGRESSIVE RELAXATION

Place yourself in a comfortable position in your chair, feet flat on the floor and hands resting comfortably in your lap. Close your eyes and take a nice, deep, relaxing breath. Focus your attention on your feet; become aware of the sensations there. You might notice that they feel different than usual—or that you can hardly feel them at all. Let those muscles relax and become soft; if you like you can even wiggle your toes and then let them rest comfortably in your shoes. Let that softness spread up into your ankles and calves. Let your lower legs be soft and as relaxed as possible. Let that softness spread up into your thighs, let your thighs be soft and relaxed. As you relax you might notice that your body feels heavier or lighter, or warmer or cooler. Whatever you feel, allow those sensations to indicate to you that you are getting more and more relaxed. Let your pelvis relax and the muscles you sit on. As you do you might notice that you sink even more deeply into the chair. Let your abdomen relax and soften and let that softness spread up into your chest and lower and midback. Take a nice deep breath and allow all those muscles to become even more soft, more relaxed, and at ease. Let your upper back and shoulders rest and become softer and more relaxed. Drop your shoulders and, when you do, you might experience the weight of your arms helping you to relax even more deeply. Let your arms relax all the way down to your hands. You might even feel the relaxation spread down and into your hands pushing tension out through your finger tips. Notice the sensations in your hands or if they feel numb note that and find it interesting that you have discovered something new. Focus again on your shoulders and let them soften again. Soften your neck and let yourself become aware of the heaviness of your head. Let all the muscles up the back of your head and into your forehead relax and become softer and softer. Let your eyes and cheeks relax. Let your jaw soften, your tongue and throat. Enjoy the pleasant sense of softness and relaxation.

GUIDED IMAGERY

Comment

Have the client get into a relaxed state and close his/her eyes. Many scenes are available to choose from: the beach, a spring day in a meadow, a cabin in the snow, floating on a pond, etc.

Forest in the Fall

Imagine that you are walking through a beautiful wood in the fall of the year. The air has just recently turned crisp and cool. It's a comfortable and invigorating temperature. It smells fresh and clean. As you walk the leaves crunch under foot. The leaves this particular fall are especially beautiful—their colors vibrant in the trees above your head. It is restful; the sunlight plays through the trees making lovely patterns of light and patches of blue sky shine above the tree tops. It is quiet except for the pleasant sound of the breezes blowing through the pine trees and a distant brook babbling. If you like, head toward that brook following the sound until you have arrived. The water sparkles in the sun. It is fresh, cold water from the mountains. If you like, you can taste the fresh cold water. Rest by the stream enjoying the pleasant scene. After a while, get up and stretch. As you move on, the trees become less dense and, finally you exit from the woods. Before you is a lush green meadow and off in the distance, fields and rolling hills. Take a nice deep breath, allowing yourself to feel rested, relaxed, and restored.

REPETITIVE MONOTONOUS TALKING
WITH EYE CLOSURE

Get into a comfortable position and find a point to look at slightly above your head. Look at that point without blinking and when your eyes get tired let them close. That's good, just keep looking at that point until your eyes get tired and then feel perfectly comfortable about closing your eyes. As you close them, allow yourself to get very deeply relaxed, deeply relaxed; that's it, deeper and deeper relaxed. Breathing easy and regularly, easy and regularly, as you get deeper and deeper relaxed. Just let yourself get as deeply relaxed as you need to be, as deeply relaxed as you need to be. Breathing in and out, in and out, that's good; softer and easier, softer and easier, more and more relaxed.

Comment

The goal of this kind of induction is to be boring and rhythmically repetitive. Breathing in rhythm with the patient and talking in that rhythm can be helpful. If the patient does not close his or her eyes, simply interpret that it's OK and if at any time he or she wants to close eyes for additional comfort that will be OK, too. The purpose is to use what is presented positively and to follow the patient's lead in making suggestions.

DEEPENING TECHNIQUES

Many techniques exist for promoting or enhancing the trance state including:

1. Counting backwards or forwards with the suggestion that on each count the individual will get more relaxed or more deeply into trance.
2. Silence.
3. Repeating phrases over and over—"deeper and deeper relaxed."
4. Imagining a descent (e.g., elevator, staircase) on each step or floor the therapist suggests that the individual get deeper relaxed or more deeply into trance.
5. A Mantra—encouraging the individual to repeat a word or a sound.
6. A cue for deepening—again a word or a sound that the individual learns to associate with the trance state.

ONE METHOD FOR TRAINING IN AUTOHYPNOSIS WITH INSTRUCTIONS FOR DEHYPNOSIS*

Comment

Begin by selecting a quiet place to spend an uninterrupted half-hour a day practicing autohypnosis. Seat yourself in a comfortable chair with your hands resting on your lap and your feet on the floor or on a foot stool. Fix your eyes on a spot on the ceiling above the level of your eyes. Take a very deep breath and blow it out very slowly as you begin to relax yourself. Focus your attention to your eyelids now and say, "Relaxation will begin now,"—and between numbers, say to yourself repeatedly that your eyes are becoming very, very tired. Say over and over, "My lids are becoming so heavy. I feel as if I want to close my eyes at the count of three. My lids are becoming heavier and heavier, now . . . they are so heavy, so very heavy; I feel that the heavier they become, the more relaxed I will become and the better able I will be to follow all

---

*Edited; original supplied by Barbara J. Smith.

suggestions I give myself. With each breath I take, the more relaxed I will feel. Now that my lids have become so very heavy, it is going to be a great pleasure to close my eyes."

Feel the heaviness of your eyelids. Let your eyes roll up with the back of your head for a few seconds. Then say, "My eyelids are closed and locked tightly together, tight, tight, tight. My lids are locked so tight, and the tighter they become the more relaxed I will become. With each breath I take, the deeper relaxed I will feel.

As a deepening technique, imagine great waves of relaxation running from the top of your head over into your body, over you and through you, one wave after the other, waves and waves of relaxation helping you relax, you are becoming very, very relaxed, your forehead relaxed, shoulders, upper arms, forearms, every muscle in your body soft and relaxed and heavy, heavy, very heavy. One wave after another, you feel almost as if the tension is flowing out of you through the tips of your fingers and the tips of your toes, waves of relaxation, draining every bit of tension out of you. All of the tension and stress in your body is slowly pouring out of your fingers and toes into the air around you, leaving nothing behind but peaceful relaxation; just relax, your muscles are soft and relaxed.

Do not get upset if you forget the exact words when you are using autohypnosis, but you may take your own tape of your voice if you like. They are far less important than the effect that you are trying to achieve.

Stay in this state until you are ready to self-dehypnotize. Remember, the next time you wish to hypnotize yourself or be hypnotized you will find it much easier; you will go much deeper and very much faster using a shorter induction. No one will ever be able to hypnotize you unless you give your verbal permission. It will be necessary for you to say aloud that you wish to be hypnotized unless you are using autohypnosis.

Now that you have relaxed for about a half hour, prepare yourself for self-dehypnosis. Say, "I will be alert, relaxed, and feeling much calmer and more able to deal with stressful encounters in a more relaxed manner in my everyday environment and work after using autohypnosis."

Count backwards from ten to one. At the count of five, your eyes will open and at the count of one, you will be fully alert and feeling calm and relaxed. Say, "ten . . . nine . . . eight . . . seven . . . six . . . five, eyes open . . . four . . . three . . . two . . . one, alert, calm, relaxed."

ARM LEVITATION

Comment

This is a standard induction used by many therapists and clinicians. Its drawback is that something specific must happen for the patient to feel successful unless the clinician reinterprets the results if the arm does not elevate. The editor suggests this technique be used by more experienced clinicians following a relaxation procedure.

INDUCTION PROCESS.   Now that you are relaxed and comfortable imagine that a string is tied around your wrist. Attached to that string is a bright red balloon filled with helium. It's a big balloon and very light and it's tugging gently on your wrist. As it tugs you may notice that your hand is getting lighter and lighter, lighter. As it becomes lighter and lighter your hand will effortlessly leave your lap and elevate ever so slowly. Up! Up! Lighter and lighter. (These suggestions are repeated and if only a finger moves the therapist can comment on that encouraging the patient that he or she is doing very well). As your hand has now elevated, let that be a signal to you to get even more deeply relaxed and comfortable.

DISCUSSION.   If the hand does not elevate simply encourage the patient to experience the pleasant feelings he or she is experiencing and to become even more deeply relaxed. If the hand lifts it can be left elevated for the remainder or allowed to drop naturally back into the lap. The return of the hand to the lap can signal a deeper state or be used in the process of dehypnotization. Prior to 'awakening' or returning to usual consciousness the therapist suggests that all normal sensations return to the hand as some numbness is commonly associated with the levitation.

ADDITIONAL ERICKSONIAN HYPNOTIC TECHNIQUES

1.   *Truisms* are simple undeniable statements about behavior that the person has either experienced or is experiencing now. The statements, because they are so obviously true, are connected to other suggestions for promoting a receptive accepting state of mind. These are often part of *contingent* and *conjunctive* suggestions and for obtaining a *yes set*, an agreeable state established by a set of obvious questions, e.g., "you do want to be more comfortable and relaxed, don't you?" (see chapter 3, p. 48).

EXAMPLES: "You woke up this morning."
"You are sitting in that chair."
"You are breathing in and out and your feet are resting on the floor."

2.   *Implied Directives* are time bound, implied, or assumed suggestions for a behavioral response.

EXAMPLES: *"When you sit in that chair and are comfortable . . .* you might begin to notice increased comfort."

>*"I'm not sure when your eyes will close* . . . but when they do
>you can become even more relaxed."
>*"Some time soon you may discover how you can use these learn-*
>*ings* . . . to begin to eat normally and moderately.

3. ***Reframing*** is changing the meaning or perception of a situation in this context so it can be viewed more positively. Reframing a situation often causes a shift in attention and perception.

EXAMPLES: ● A crisis can be seen as an opportunity for growth. The symbol for *crisis* in Chinese means opportunity.
● When a wound begins to itch it means it is healing.
● Rather than describing an overweight person as obese, use *zaftig*, volumptuous, hefty, or substantial.

4. ***Double Bind*** is a technique that suggests the same end result but with different means to obtain that result or that the person use the same desired means to different ends. The primary goal of some change in the client, however, is kept consistent.

EXAMPLES: "I don't know which arm will become more relaxed and begin to lift first—your right arm or your left arm."
"I don't know when you will stop smoking—today or tomorrow."
"You can discover either how to relax or ways to be less tense by practicing relaxation techniques."

INDIRECT ERICKSONIAN HYPNOTIC INDUCTION

This example is written for a preoperative patient (explanation in italics).

(Conversational tone) It is very interesting how people recently have been learning stress management techniques and applying them to many things. For example, by practicing relaxation, they are learning to reduce blood pressure. Some people even think it helps the immune system function more efficiently. I know someone who got out of the hospital much sooner and had much more postoperative comfort than he expected as a result of practicing self-hypnosis, imagery, and relaxation.

(The above is telling a story, setting the stage, and relating the use of trance to several desired ends: postoperative comfort, leaving the hospital sooner, and adequate immune functioning for healing.)

I wonder which technique will help you the most *(double bind since all the techniques are similar)* How about starting with some nice relaxing? Allow your body, as you are breathing in and out, to become more relaxed with each breath you take *(contingent suggestion)*. There may be parts of your body that get more relaxed than others and you may also note that different parts of your body feel different *(dissociation)* as you are relaxing more and more. It can be so nice to relax and we know it can be so good for you. Don't you agree that feeling relaxed is certainly more pleasant and comfortable than feeling stressed and tense? *(yes set)* I'm not sure when you will feel the increased comfort with the relaxation *(open-ended suggestion)*, but comfort and calm can be such a nice part of breathing more regularly. You can even count to yourself if that seems to help and if it produces a nice sense of distraction and more comfort *(future-oriented suggestion tied to self hypnosis techniques)*. And your unconscious and conscious mind can both always remember times when you felt very comfortable, and those feelings of comfort and relaxation can be recaptured when you remember those times. Those feelings and memories can be so helpful in your healing and recovery . . .

Additional Readings

Barber, J. and Adrian, C. (1982). *Psychological approaches to the management of pain.* New York: Brunner/Mazel, Inc.

Barker, P. (1985). *Using metaphors in psychotherapy.* New York: Brunner/Mazel, Inc.

Borysenko, J. (1987). *Minding the body; mending the mind.* New York: Bantam Books.

Carson, R. (1983). *Taming your gremlin; A guide to enjoy yourself.* New York: Harper and Row.

Crasilneck, H.B. and Hall, J.A. (1985). *Clinical hypnosis: Principles and applications,* 2nd ed. Orlando, FL: Grune and Stratton, Inc.

Citrenbaum, C.M., King, M.E., and Cohen, W.I. (1985). *Modern clinical hypnosis for habit control.* New York: W.W. Norton, Co.

Dolan, Y. (1985). *A path with a heart: Ericksonian utilization with resistant and chronic patients.* New York: Brunner/Mazel, Inc.

Dowd, T.E. and Healy, J.M. (1986). *Case studies in hypnotherapy.* New York: Guilford Publishers.

Erickson, M. (Eds. E.L. Rossi and M.O. Ryan) (1985). *Life reframing in hypnosis: The seminars, workshops and lectures of Milton H. Erickson. Vol II.* New York: Irvington Publishers.

Erickson, M. (Eds. E.L. Rossi and M.O. Ryan) (1986). *Mind body communication in hypnosis: The seminars, workshops and lectures of Milton H. Erickson. Vol III.* New York: Irvington Publishers.

Havens, R.A. and Walters, C. (1989). *Hypnotherapy scripts: A neo-ericksonian approach to persuasive healing.* New York: Brunner/Mazel, Inc.

Hoorwitz, A.N. (1989). *Hypnotic methods in non-hypnotic therapies.* New York: Irvington Publishers.

Lankton, S. and Lankton, C. (1983). *The answer within: A clinical framework of Ericksonian hypnotherapy.* New York: Brunner/Mazel, Inc.

Lankton S. and Lankton C. (1989). *Tales of enchantment: Goal oriented metaphors for adults and children in therapy.* New York: Brunner/Mazel, Inc.

Mills, J.C. and Crowley, R.J. (1986). *Therapeutic metaphors for children and the child within.* New York: Brunner/Mazel, Inc.

O'Hanlon, W.H. (1987). *Taproots: Underlying principles of Milton Erickson's therapy and hypnosis.* New York: W.W. Norton Co.

Rossi, E. (1986). *Psychobiology of mind-body healing: New concepts of therapeutic hypnosis.* New York: W.W. Norton Co.

Rossi, E.L. and Cheek D.B. (1988). *Mind-body therapy: Methods of ideodynamic healing in hypnosis.* New York: W.W. Norton, Co.

Rosen, S. (Ed.) (1982). *My voice will go with you: The teaching tales of Milton H. Erickson.* New York: W.W. Norton, Co.

Soskis, D. (1986). *Teaching self hypnosis: An introductory guide for clinicians.* New York: W.W. Norton, Co.

Steffenhagen, R.A. (Ed.) (1983). *Hypnotic techniques for increasing self esteem.* New York: Irvington Publishers.

Wallas, L. (1985). *Stories for the third ear: Using hypnotic fables in psychotherapy.* New York: W.W. Norton Co.

Wester, W.C. II and Smith, H. Jr. (Eds.) (1984). *Clinical hypnosis: A multidisciplinary approach.* Philadelphia, PA: J.B. Lippincott Co.

Wright, E.M. and Wright, B.A. (1987). *Clinical practice of hypnotherapy.* New York: Guilford Publishing.

Yapko, M.D. (1990). *Trancework: An introduction to the practice of clinical hypnosis.* New York: Brunner/Mazel, Inc.

Zahourek, R.P. (Ed.) (1988). *Relaxation and imagery: Tools of therapeutic communication and intervention.* Philadelphia, PA: W.B. Saunders Co.

Zilbergeld, B., Edelstein, M.G., & Araoz, D.L. (Eds.) (1986). *Hypnosis: Questions and Answers.* New York: W.W. Norton Co.

Zeig, J. and Lankton, S.R. (1988). *Developing ericksonian therapy: State of the Art.* New York: Brunner/Mazel, Inc.

Index

Contributors

Susan Plock Bromley, M.S.W., Psy.D. Assistant Professor of Psychology, University of Northern Colorado, Greeley, Colorado

Carolyn Chambers Clark, R.N., Ed.D., F.A.A.N. Editor/Publisher *The Wellness Newsletter*; Nursing Consultant, VA Hospital, Bay Pines, Florida

Marcia G. Fishman, R.N., M.A. Lecturer, Private Practice, Counseling in Thanatology, New York, New York

Maureen Shawn Kennedy, R.N., M.A. Consultant, Convention Manager, American Journal of Nursing Company, New York, New York

Jeanine L. LaBaw, R.N., M.S., Psy.D. Private Practice, Denver, Colorado

Wallace L. LaBaw, M.D., F.R.S.H. Child Psychiatrist, Private Practice; Volunteer Faculty, Health Sciences Center, University of Colorado, Denver, Colorado

Dorothy Marie Larkin, M.A., R.N. Adjunct Faculty Graduate Nursing Program, College of New Rochelle, New York; Consultant Cabrini Hospice, New York

Ronald L. McBride, B.S.N., C.R.N.A., C.N. Assistant Director, Graduate Program in Nurse Anesthesiology, Baylor College of Medicine, Houston, Texas

Louis R. McCoy, R.N., Ph.D., C.R.N.A. Founder and Former Director, American Academy of Clinical Hypnosis; Former Dean, American College of Hypnotherapy, New Orleans, Louisiana

Stanley Meyers, Ph.D. Director of Clinical Training Center for the Advancement of Group Studies, New York, New York

Eileen O'Connell, R.N., M.S. Private Practice, Psychotherapy for Adults and Children, West Roxbury, Massachusetts

Barbara J. Smith, R.N., M.S.N. Administrative Coordinator of Hospital Liaison, Psychiatric Service, Maimonides Community Mental Medical Center, Brooklyn, New York

Marie Stoner, M.Ed. Psychologist in Private Practice; Lecturer, Thomas Jefferson University, Philadelphia, Pennsylvania

Rothlyn P. Zahourek, M.S., R.N., C.S. Private Psychotherapy and Consultation Practice, Amherst, Massachusetts